SRI AUROBINDO AND HIS YOGA

M.P. PANDIT

PUBLISHER:
LOTUS LIGHT PUBLICATIONS
P.O. Box 2
Wilmot, WI 53192 U.S.A.

CONTENTS

Part I: Sri Aurobindo: A Survey

Part II: Sadhana in Sri Aurobindo's Yoga

SRI AUROBINDO
AND
HIS YOGA

PART I
Sri Aurobindo: A Survey

SRI AUROBINDO

Reacting to the importunities of biographers, Sri Aurobindo once remarked that none could write on his life for it was not there on the surface for man to see. And that in spite of the spectacular roles played by him in the different spheres of life. What was he really? A poet? For, apart from the large number of sonnets, lyrics, poetical plays, poems from the surrealist to the mystic, he has given us the longest epic in English verse, *Savitri, a legend and a symbol*. A statesman? Was it not he who gave a clear political ideal to the resurgent India, channelised the nationalist aspirations into an effective revolutionary movement and set the country on the road to complete freedom? Has he not developed the ideal of nationalism into the greater ideal of Human Unity and established its inevitability in the mind of man through his prophetic writings? A philosopher? Has he not presented the grand philosophy of *Life Divine* which unites in its sweep both the ends of existence, the Spirit and Matter, which have hitherto defied reconciliation and kept man and God apart? Has he not perceived a definite meaning and direction in the life-movement, whether individual or universal, pointing to the truth of a spiritual evolution? A mystic? Who can surpass the spiritual realisations and the soul-experience and the rising curves of Consciousness that transcend the limits of logical reason recorded by him in his innumerable writings on yoga? And there are other personalities that claim our attention. But first let

us have a look at the most external details of his
career that provide the framework as it were for his
multi-faceted life.

Sri Aurobindo was born in Calcutta on August 15,
1872. He was born in an aristocracy of culture; his
maternal grandfather was the much-respected Raj-
narayan Bose, a leader of the Indian Renaissance of
that age. His father, Dr. Krishna Dhan Ghose, was a
popular civil surgeon and a centre of cultural life
wherever he was posted. At the age of five, Aurobindo
was sent to a Convent school in Darjeeling and two
years later taken to England for his education. He was
left with a private family at Manchester for his education and upbringing with the instructions that he
should be given a completely English education. Sri
Aurobindo was there in England for 14 years during
which he acquired great proficiency in the classical
languages, Latin and Greek, and learnt a number of
continental languages too. He wrote poetry, won all the
prizes that were open to him and distinguished himself
both at St. Paul's School and at Cambridge where he
studied. He devoted more time for extracurricular
studies than to class-books. His father had desired him
to pass the I. C. S. examination and accordingly young
Aurobindo passed the written examination. But having
no interest in the career held forth by the I. C. S. he
got himself disqualified by failing to appear for the
riding test. There was another reason why he was not
keen on joining this Service. The winds of unrest in
India against the alien British rule had blown over his

soul and he had a presentiment that he was to play a definite part in the political emancipation of his country. He even made some fiery speeches in the Indian Majlis at Cambridge on this subject.

Though he was, thus, not admitted into the Indian Civil Service, circumstances favoured him with an appointment from the Gaikwad, ruler of Baroda State, who was then on a visit to England. Sri Aurobindo sailed for India in 1893 with this appointment in his pocket. The return of this unique son to her bosom was greeted by Mother India in a memorable manner. As soon as Sri Aurobindo stepped on the Indian soil at Apollo Bunder, a vast Calm descended upon him and continued to be with him for a long time after. From Bombay he proceeded to Baroda where he spent the next fourteen years of his life, in various positions — in the Secretariat, in the palace of the Maharaja, in the College first as a professor and then as the vice-Principal. Side by side with his official duties, he pursued his own studies in Indian scriptures and classics in order to acquaint himself with the genuine Indian tradition at first hand. He also learnt important modern Indian languages like Gujarati, Marathi and Bengali. He read widely and many of his literary works were really begun — some of them completed — during this period. Especially some of his plays and narrative poems were done in these years. Sri Aurobindo had a close look at the political situation in the country in the very beginning of his stay at Baroda. He wrote a series of articles entitled "New Lamps for Old" condemning the mendi-

cant mentality of the Congress leadership of that time
and calling for a more energetic approach. He also
interested himself in the revolutionary movements that
were germinating in several parts of the country and
established contacts with some of them. His official
position did not allow him to participate openly in the
nationalist movement. That is why he worked from behind the scenes for a long time and took the plunge
only when the situation was ripe for a bold action.

That occasion was provided by the crisis over the
Bengal partition enactment and Sri Aurobindo assumed
leadership of the extremist section of the movement.
He wrote fiery articles in the famous *Bande Mataram*
journal and awakened the whole country to the
urgency of concerted action to win complete independence for India. His programme was two-edged: nega-
tively boycott and non-co-operation, positively, swadeshi
and national regeneration. There was a revolutionary
side to this movement to which Sri Aurobindo lent his
support but he sought to harness the revolutionary fervour
of the youth to the spiritual ideal of the Motherhood
of India. The British Government foisted a case and
kept him in jail for one full year. It was during this
incarceration that Sri Aurobindo had the realisation of
Vasudeva as the one Lord of the Universe and His
Consciousness as the stuff of the world. Sri Aurobindo
was shown a wider vista than the national field and
given a glimpse of a larger work awaiting him. As
assured from within, Sri Aurobindo was acquitted after
a historic trial and memorable defence by C. R. Das

in 1909. When Sri Aurobindo came out of jail he found that repression had temporarily broken the spirit of the general nationalist movement, the leaders were removed from the scene and a spirit of depression prevailed. Valiantly he undertook to arouse his countrymen and for this purpose started two Journals, the *Karmayogin* in English and *Dharma* in Bengali in which he recalled to his fellowmen the fundamental values of their ancient heritage, explained their duty to their motherland and to their posterity. He toured the districts of Bengal and spoke widely on his programme. But he clearly saw that the movement he had started had to take a different shape and he was not to be the leader. He received an Adesh, a divine command, from above to proceed to Chandernagore, a French possession near Calcutta. He obeyed instantly and arrived in Chandernagore incognito, where he stayed for about a month before he was guided to proceed to Pondicherry, the destined place for the real mission for which he was born.

He arrived in Pondicherry with one or two companions on the 4th April, 1910. He settled down with the help of the local gentry in private lodgings and slowly switched over his active interest from the political to a spiritual sphere. Sri Aurobindo's turning to the spiritual side of life was, however, not sudden. Even when he was a boy in England he had glimpses of a life greater than the ordinary physical existence with which most men are preoccupied. When he was reading Max Muller's translation of the Upanishads he had a distinct experience of the Self. We have already referred to the descent of a supernatural Calm on him on his return to India. While at Baroda his interest in yoga was awakened — not for personal salvation but for gaining irresistible power for the liberation of the motherland, and with the help of a friend he started *prāṇāyāma*. He records in one of his letters that though no spiritual progress was seen by this exercise, certain other faculties developed and he was able to write poetry for hours together with a speed that was amazing. However, he came into contact with a Maharashtrian yogi, Vishnu Bhaskar Lele, and he was given a method of communing with the Divine seated within the heart and surrendering to Him. Apart from his efforts in this direction, he was vouchsafed experiences of the vision of the Godhead when once in danger, the infinity of Brahman while in Kashmir. All these movements received a decisive confirmation during his stay in the Alipore jail in Calcutta where he had a series of experiences culminating in the realisation of the cosmic consciousness. What happened later in Pondicherry is a separate chapter to which we shall presently turn.

At Pondicherry Sri Aurobindo devoted himself exclusively to yoga, not to any of the well-trodden older yogas but to a new line of yoga which was gradually revealing itself to him. Glimpses of the goal of this yoga are indeed there in his writings in the *Karma-yogin*, especially his renderings of the Isha and the Kena Upanishads. His was the path of affirmation, fulfilment of the Divine in this world which is His manifestation. Life is the field of this revelation of God and should be accepted as such. The object of human existence is to realise the divinity of man in a world essentially divine. This vision of truth is veiled by a thick crust of ignorance and yoga is the means to break through this crust and realise the true character of life. Sri Aurobindo pursued his effort in this untrodden direction and started the journal *Arya* in 1914 by which time he was in full possession of the Knowledge he was seeking and had a clear perception of the world to come. In this monthly, Sri Aurobindo expounded his metaphysic of *The Life Divine*, presenting a full-fledged philosophy of an Omnipresent Reality, the Destiny of man, the Goal of Spiritual Evolution and the inevitability of a divine life for the most evolved. He wrote another series entitled *The Synthesis of Yoga* in which he summed up the contribution of the past methods of yoga and outlined his own yoga of self-perfection for realising the ideal of the Life Divine. He studied the sociological and the political development of humanity in the light of this perception of spiritual evolution and oneness of origin in the Divine and wrote at length on *The Psychology of Social Development* (now published as *The Human Cycle*) and *The Ideal of Human Unity*. He delved into the Indian scriptures to see whether the ancient wisdom corroborated his own realisation of the truth of divine manifestation in the world through a spiritual evolution of consciousness and he embodied the results of his enquiry in his *Secret of the Veda, Hymns to the Mystic Fire,* Commentaries on the *Upa-*

nishads and *Essays on the Gita*. Poet that he was, he was interested in the role of the potent word, *mantra*, in the evolution of literary expression; *The Future Poetry* was the result.

Sri Aurobindo wrote almost all the 64 pages of the *Arya* every month by himself and carried on the project for six and a half years till 1921. The profundity and the range of knowledge formulated in the writings in the *Arya* is something phenomenal. Yet Sri Aurobindo once observed that he had revealed in the *Arya* only a fraction of the Knowledge that came to him in his *tapasya*.

All these years, though he was primarily concerned with the spiritual side of life and was engaged in devoloping an integral system of yoga to reach the goal of the integral perfection of man in God and for God in this world, he continued to take interest in the political and connected events in India and elsewhere. He was again and again pressed by the leaders of the Indian National Congress to return to the political scene and guide the country. However, he declined repeatedly saying that he no more believed in the human methods of the day but was in search of an unfailing divine Power which could be man's if only he developed himself into the necessary consciousness to wield it. He believed that the present state of imperfection, ego-ridden, divided in being and maimed in power is not the final stage of human evolution. He saw that the next stage in the evolution of man is to grow into a consciousness beyond the limited mentality that is his today. He permitted those who accepted this Ideal to share this knowledge with him and practise the yoga developed by him under his guidance.

Slowly an Ashram grew up around him. It was in November 1926 that he retired into complete seclusion for a more intensive pursuit of his yoga, leaving the entire charge of the Ashram in the hands of the Mother, his radiant collaborator. Though the Ashram then had hardly a score of disciples, it represented an experiment in collective living dedicated to a common spiritual ideal and it held out many significant possibilities towards the realisation of an eventual Gnostic community. We will have occasion to refer to the subsequent growth of the Ashram elsewhere. Suffice it to say that Sri Aurobindo identified himself with the aspirations and struggles of the seekers that gathered in the Ashram from all parts of the world, bore their burden and made their path towards the Light easier till the very last moment of his physical life on earth in December 1950.

Sri Aurobindo gave a positive Ideal of Perfection to humanity. His message has given hope to the meanest of the creatures on earth. Life has been elevated to a divine value. Man no more dreams but is on the way to becoming a god. And more.

SRI AUROBINDO'S PHILOSOPHY

Sri Aurobindo does not think or build in vacuum. His philosophy is not something that is woven in the flights of speculative intellect. It is based on the solid foundations of his spiritual experience ripening into realisation. He takes care to verify this experience with reference to past spiritual realisations and see how far they corroborate his line of experience and the Vision that he sees, *darśana*. Not that he is content to merely restate the past gains in his own terms; he allows the experience to develop naturally and records what he realises, reasons it out for presentation to the logical mind, relating it to the whole movement of humanity.

Sri Aurobindo is at one with the perception of the Rishis of the Upanishad that man is essentially divine. He points out, however, that this truth of the Upanishad, *tat tvam asi,* Thou art That, has not been sufficiently understood in the light of the other statement, *sarvam khalu idam brahma*, All this is Brahman. Not merely you or I, but the whole of the universe is Brahman. Yes, Brahman is all this: there is naught else in creation but Brahman. It is in this sense that his philosophy is called realistic *advaita*.

Far-reaching consequences follow from this basic conception. The world-movement acquires a significance as a willed manifestation of Brahman, the Divine. It is not just a play, not a seeming operation, but a movement with a purpose. There is an Intelligence that is behind every movement in the universe, *prajñā netro lokah.* And that Intelligence is none other than the Divine Consciousness itself, *prajnanam brahma.*

Life is a field for the manifestation of the Divine Consciousness. In all forms, in all movements, there is a consciousness that is trying to express itself, organise itself and develop itself. This is both on the microcosmic and the macrocosmic levels. Evolution, spiritual evolution, is the method by which the element of consciousness that is ingrained in every form seeks to grow and take full shape. The history of the Earth is verily a history of the evolution of this involved consciousness.

From arid Matter, nescient and inert, breaks out the first stirring of consciousness in sensations of life. Life gradually develops, takes shape and when sufficiently organised, it shows rudiments of mental awareness and intelligence. Mind begins to form itself. Evolution is really this phenomenon of the growth of consciousness; development of forms on which Darwin and other evolutionists lay so much stress is only the external process of Nature which strives to forge forms appropriate to the state of consciousness developed. The consciousness determines the form.

The evolution of the Earth has registered three well-marked stages — Matter, Life, Mind. Mark, that all these are formulations of the Divine Consciousness for the purpose of manifestation; they too are, each, Brahman: *annam brahma, prāno brahma, mano brahma.* Man, the mental purusha, is the highest type so far evolved on earth in this general progression. But this is not the end. Mind is not the last word. It is too limited a form, too scanty a light to be the crown of the age-long effort of Nature. Beyond the Mind is the Spirit, the spiritual Purusha, the Divine Consciousness organised as the faculty of Knowledge-Will, the Vijnana. It is a principle of Truth as Knowledge infallible and Power unfailing, existing on a level beyond the mind — the supermind. To realise and embody on earth this Power of the supramental Truth is the next stage of Evolution. The supermind marks both the culmination of the mind and its transcendence. It is a self-effective Force of Harmony, Oneness, Right and Truth which, when realised and made a part of life, can alter the whole character of existence.

If the world is the field of this evolutionary manifestation of the Spirit, the individual is the centre and the means. He is the self-aware instrument of the ordained Process. The individual who is awakened to the imperfect nature of his life, who feels the irresistible urge to break out of the limitations of desire, incapacity and death that riddle his existence, proceeds, by some means or other, to enlarge his awareness, the scope and power of his consciousness, to acquire new dimensions to his life and build in himself a new nature, a new centre of functioning; he shifts his focus from the exterior to the interior, from *bahirmukha* to *antarmukha*. In a word he does Yoga.

By self-discipline and concentration of his energies, *tapasyā*, it is possible for man to bring into operation larger and greater faculties of his being into his life.

He becomes conscious of the soul within himself, the veritable portion of the Divine at the core of his being, *mamaivaṁśaḥ*; the human personality is slowly changed and changed into the nature of the divine Person within. He opens up ranges above the active mind and is overwhelmed by the many ranges of consciousnesses that are activised — those of spontaneous thought-knowledge, of illumination, of intuition, of revelation. He is flooded by a downpour of Peace, of Power, of Light. The mental consciousness is being replaced by the supramental consciousness. Man is on his way to becoming the superman.

SRI AUROBINDO'S YOGA

Yoga is a specialised intensification of the process of Nature. Nature strives to develop the evolving consciousness and build suitable forms to embody the various types of consciousness developed by her. She has her own large ways of doing it; comprehensiveness rather than speed is her mode of working. Yoga takes up the process consciously, accelerates it and aims to arrive at the fullest development of the being within a comparatively short period. For that purpose it selects any one faculty that is more ready in the individual, viz, the mind, the emotions, the life-force, the physical body, and concentrates on developing it to its utmost potentialities, on perfecting it in its divine term. The yoga is named according to the objective and the instrument chosen for the change, viz, Jnana Yoga, Bhakti Yoga, Karma Yoga, Raja Yoga, etc. Each aims to liberate one strong part and through it to communicate the gains to the rest of the being as far as possible. One part purified and divinised (or at least spiritualised) acts as the door for the soul to free itself from the hold of Ignorance. This is the general principle stated in its broad bearings.

Sri Aurobindo's yoga aims at the liberation and *perfection* of not any one part alone, but of the whole of the being of man. It takes up all nature for the necessary transformation; its approach is integral, its goal is integral and hence its means too are integral. His is the Integral Yoga, *pūrṇa-yoga*.

One may start at any point, but as the yoga takes shape, all the faculties of the being are gathered up, brought into a focus and offered to the Divine Shakti for its transforming action. All are necessary: knowledge, devotion, powers of life, and care is taken to open oneself on all these levels. Aspiration for the divine life, surrender to the Divine, rejection of all that stands in the way of this surrender and aspiration, are the main ways. There are three great steps which mark the progression of this yoga.

The first stage in the sadhana is to become aware of the divine Person within oneself. At the core of the being, in the centre of the spiritual heart is the psychic being, the soul in evolution, a portion of the Divine. By concentration, meditation, prayer, one becomes increasingly aware of this veiled divinity, establishes contact with it and by a discipline of purification, subtlisation and consecration attains identity with it. But the integral yogin is not satisfied with this realisation of union with the Individual Divine in the depths of his being. He makes that the effective centre of his life-movements, influences and casts them in its image. He psychicises his nature. This culmination of the first stage marks the beginning of the second.

His realisation of the Divine in himself is not complete unless it is extended into a realisation of the Divine in others, in the universe around. He enlarges his vision, his mental and spiritual horizons, wider and still wider till he embraces in his consciousness the All. He perceives and lives in the consciousness of others with all. Unity, Harmony and Oneness of Origin in the Divine are self-evident truths to him. He has arrived at the realisation of the Cosmic Divine which in turn points to the next, the third culmination.

The unitive realisation has been extended horizontally into the Universal. But both of them derive their truth from another, the Transcendent which has formulated itself in them both. And unless this Transcendent Divine which is not subject to the conditions of the individual and the universal formulations is realised, the liberation is not complete. This goal is reached through a series of openings upwards in the being, to ranges of consciousness that extend higher and higher above the mind and constitute the *parārdha* the upper hemisphere above the triple Ignorance of mind-life-body.

A capital step in the ascension is the realisation of a Truth-Consciousness called Ritam in the Veda, Vijnana in the Upanishads, the Mahas in later texts, the Supramental Consciousness in Sri Aurobindo's philosophy. To arrive at this consciousness of Truth-Will and establish it in oneself is the final aim set before the sadhaka in this yoga. This is the faculty of consciousness above the highest levels of the Mind to which human evolution unmistakably points. For only such a Truth-principle as this can eliminate the imperfections to which man has been subject due to the hold of Ignorance, and establish the reign of the divine verities, Truth in place of Ignorance, Power in place of limitation, Bliss in place of Pain, Immortality in place of Death.

SRI AUROBINDO ON THE VEDA

Sri Aurobindo studied the Veda, Upanishads and the Gita not with a view to interpret them in the light of any philosophy formulated by his mind but in order to see what corroboration they offered to the body of spiritual experience that had grown in himself during the years of his concentrated *tapasya*.

His entry into the Veda was in a way accidental. Much was being talked of in those days regarding the alleged invasion by the Aryans of a Dravidian India in ages gone by, the historical enmity between the two distinct races and so on. Curious to know what the old hymns of the Veda had to say on the point, Sri Aurobindo took up the Rig Veda for study. Soon, however, he was obliged to leave the starting-point of his interest and pursue certain other lines of thought and psychological experiences that opened up to his vision in those hymns. For, he perceived there an arrangement of certain Deities that corresponded with his own realisations in Yoga. This fact led him deeper and in directions other than what he had expected.

His studies revealed that the ritualistic content of the Veda so ably upheld by Sayana and other commentators of his persuasion and the naturalistic character highlighted by Western scholars were only the outer frames, external aspects of a conserved body of spiritual knowledge and experience of the ancients. Behind the deceptive exterior there lay a profound corpus of the history and record of the inner communion of the Rishis —

leaders of the Aryan society in that age — and the Gods, Powers of the creative Godhead. The outer ritual was throughout paralleled by an inner process of self-consecration and self-giving to the higher Divine Powers of the Cosmos. Sri Aurobindo recalled the weighty statement of the old lexicographer and etymologist Yaska that the Veda has a triple meaning — ritualistic, relating to the cosmic Gods and relating to the self — the soul of man, *adhiyajña, adhideva, adhyātma*. Also Yaska's observation that roots in Sanskrit have multiple significances came as an invaluable help in understanding the hymnal at more levels than one. Sri Aurobindo announced the results of his studies in a series of essays entitled the *Secret of the Veda* and followed it up with *Selected Hymns* with commentaries illustrating and justifying his approach. The central idea, to quote rather extensively from his writings, was this:

"The hymns were written in a stage of religious culture which answered to a similar period in Greece and other ancient countries, a stage in which there was a double face to the current religion, an outer for the people, *profanum vulgus*, and inner for the initiates, the early period of the Mysteries. The Vedic Rishis were mystics who reserved their inner knowledge for the initiates; they shielded them from the vulgar by the use of an alphabet of symbols which could not readily be understood without the initiation, but were perfectly clear and systematic when the signs were once known.

"These symbols centred around the idea and forms
of the sacrifice; for the sacrifice was the universal and
central institution of the prevailing cult. The hymns
were written round this institution and were understood
by the vulgar as ritual chants in praise of the Nature
gods, — Indra, Agni, Surya, Rudra, Vishnu, Sarasvati,
with the object of provoking by the sacrifice the gifts
of the gods, — cows, horses, gold and the other forms
of wealth of a pastoral people, victory over enemies,
safety in travel, sons, servants, prosperity, every kind
of material good fortune. But behind this mask of pri-
mitive and materialistic naturalism, lay another and
esoteric cult which would reveal itself if we once pene-
trated the meaning of the Vedic symbols. That once
caught and rightly read, the whole of Rig Veda would
become clear, consequent, a finely woven, yet straightforward tissue.

"The outer sacrifice represented in these esoteric
terms an inner sacrifice of self-giving and communion
with the gods. These gods are powers, outwardly of
physical, inwardly of psychical nature. Thus, Agni
outwardly is the physical principle of fire but inwardly
the god of the psychic godward flame, force, will,
Tapas; Surya outwardly the solar light, inwardly the
god of the illuminating revelatory knowledge, Soma
outwardly the moon and the Soma wine or nectarous
moon-plant, inwardly the god of the spiritual ecstasy,
Ananda. The principal psychical conception of this
inner Vedic cult was the idea of the Satyam, Ritam,
Brihat, the Truth, the Law, the Vast. Earth, Air and

Heaven symbolised the physical, vital and mental being, but this Truth was situated in the greater heaven, base of a triple Infinity actually and explicitly mentioned in the Vedic Riks, and it meant therefore a state of spiritual and supramental illumination. To get beyond earth and sky to Svar, the Sun-world, seat of this illumination, home of the gods, foundation and seat of the Truth, was the achievement of the early Fathers, *pūrve pitaraḥ*, and of the seven Angirasa Rishis who founded the Vedic religion. The solar gods, children of Infinity, *ādityāḥ*, were born in the Truth and the Truth was their home, but they descended into the lower planes and had in each plane their appropriate functions, their mental, vital and physical cosmic motions. They were the guardians and increasers of the Truth in man and by the Truth, *ṛtasya patha*, led him to felicity and immortality. They had to be called into the human being: and increased, in their functioning formed in him, brought in or born, *devavīti*, extended, *devatāti*, united in their universality, *vaiśvadevya*.

"The sacrifice was represented at once as a giving and worship, a battle and a journey. It was the centre of a battle between the Gods aided by Aryan men on one side and the Titans or destroyers on the opposite faction, Dasyus, Vritras, Panis, Rakshasas, later called Daityas and Asuras, between the powers of falsehood, division, darkness. It was a journey, because the sacrifice travelled from earth to the gods in their heaven, but also because it made ready the path by which man himself travelled to the Home of the Truth.

This journey opposed by the Dasyus, thieves, robbers, tearers, besiegers (Vritras), was itself a battle. The giving was an inner giving. All the offerings of the outer sacrifice, the cow and its yield, the horse, the Soma were symbols of the dedication of inner powers and experiences to the Lords of Truth. The divine gifts, the cows of the divine light symbolised by the herds of the sun, the horse of strength and power, the sun of the inner godhead or divine man created by the sacrifice, and so through the whole list. This symbolic duplication was facilitated by the double meaning of the Vedic words; *go*, for instance, means both cow and ray; the cows of the dawn and the sun, Heaven's *boes Helioio*, are the rays of the sun-god, Lord of Revelation, even as in Greek mythology Apollo the sun-god is also Master of poetry and of prophecy; *ghrta* means clarified butter, but also the bright thing; *soma* means the wine of the moon-plant, but also delight, honey, sweetness, *madhu*. This is the conception, all other features are subsidiary to this central idea."

The way of the Vedic seers was thus one of positive fulfilment of life in this world. The Earth is the field of action and achievement with Nature, Man and Gods as the participants, the goal is the plenary manifestation of the Supreme Sun of Gnostic Light in humanity. Sri Aurobindo had hoped to work out this method taking up each Rik of the Rig Veda. He did so with most of the hymns to Agni, some on Indra, Soma and other deities. But other pressing preoccupations did not permit further work on the subject. However, his disciple, Sri Kapali Sastriar wrote his *Siddhānjana*, commenting on the first Ashtaka of the Rig Veda (the first Eighth) in Sanskrit along with a comprehensive introduction, closely following Sri Aurobindo's method of esoteric interpretation. This work is now being translated into English.

SRI AUROBINDO ON THE UPANISHADS

Sri Aurobindo perceives an unbroken continuity between the Veda and the Upanishad. At the decline of the Vedic Age after its full vigour of life, there was an inevitable encrustation of the mystic tradition. Soon, however, there followed a movement of revival and this took two lines of development. One took the form of the reclamation of the esoteric content of the Vedic heritage, the spiritual knowledge gained by the ancient seers. The other was concerned with the preservation of the ritualistic aspect, the externals of the Vedic Religion. The later took shape in the Brahmanas and the former in the Upanishads.

The Upanishads seek to hold and continue the mystic and spiritual experience — with the knowledge ensuing from it — recorded in the hymns of the Veda. The Rishis of this era start from the fundamental truths proclaimed in the litany and strive to realise them in their own experience. Or when they arrive at any realisation of the Supreme Truth by their own *tapasyā*, they seek confirmation from the experience of the earlier seers. Sri Aurobindo cites several instances of these exercises and describes how the cryptic contents of the hymns come in for amplified re-statement in the Upanishads, albeit in a language more suited to the mentality of a later age.

Naturally the outlook and the inlook of the Rishis of the Upanishads — at any rate of the earlier and authentic texts — is in the line of the seers of the Veda. The emphasis is on the realisation of the Truth and living it here only, *ihaiva*, not somewhere beyond after death. The world to them is a manifestation of the Divine, the Brahman, with the Gods as so many Powers and Personalities entrusted with the task of governing the universe and helping the creation — at all levels of its life — to evolve into the image of the creative Divinity and fully participate in the glory of the Manifestation. The approach is positive and comprehensive. The whole of creation is embraced in the scheme of life.

The Isha begins with the declaration that All this is for the habitation of the Lord. It describes how the universe is a Becoming of the Divine Being in His mood to manifest. It concludes emphasising the identity between man and God and shows the "straight way of the truth" to realise it in life. The Kena asks what it is that impels the eye to see, the ear to hear, the mind to hit its mark? In a word, what makes the senses reach out to and grasp the world in their experience? And it answers that there is a Master-Sense that operates through all these external faculties. This Master-Sense is a function of the Divinity manifest in the universe and it should be worshipped as Delight, *tadvanam*. Deiight is the key-note of creation and life is intended to participate in this Pure Joy by eliminating from its course all the obscuring, deflecting, depraving elements of ignorance, inertia and falsehood. The Taittiriya celebrates the pervasion of the Divine Reality at all the levels of creation from gross Matter, *annam brahma* to the Blissful Spirit, *ānandam brahma*. It describes the multiple being of man, relates it step by step to the corresponding planes of universal Existence and calls upon the seeker to concentrate his consciousness and realise this Reality integrally in the universe.

Sri Aurobindo's commentaries on the Isha and the Kena, readings in the Taittiriya, translations of Katha, Mundaka, Mandukya, Aitareya and Prashna Upanishads expound this Integral Knowledge embracing Man, Nature and God in a meaningful whole. His series on the *Philosophy of the Upanishads*, written early in his career, draw pointed attention to the fact of growing confirmation of the Vedantic truths enshrined in the Upanishads by the findings of modern Science.

To conclude in his own words:

"The Upanishads have been the acknowledged source of numerous profound philosophies and religions that flowed from it in India like her great rivers from their Himalayan cradle fertilising the mind and life of the people and kept its soul alive through the long procession of the centuries, constantly returned to for light, never failing to give fresh illumination, a fountain of inexhaustible life-giving waters. Buddhism with all its developments was only a restatement, although from a new standpoint and with fresh terms of intellectual definition and reasoning, of one side of its experience and it carried it thus changed in form but hardly in substance over all Asia and westward towards Europe. The ideas of the Upanishads can be rediscovered in much of the thought of Pythagoras and Plato and form the profoundest part of Neo-Platonism and Gnosticism with all their considerable consequences to the philosophical thinking of the West, and Sufism only repeats them in another religious language. The larger part of German metaphysics is little more in substance than an intellectual development of great realities more spiritually seen in this ancient teaching, and modern thought is rapidly absorbing them with a closer, more living and intense receptiveness which promises a revolution both in philosophical and in religious thinking; here they are filtering in through many indirect influences, there slowly pouring through direct and open channels. There is hardly a main philosophical idea which cannot find an authority or a seed or indication in these antique writings — the speculations, according to a certain view, of thinkers who had no better past or background to their thought than a crude, barbaric, naturalistic and animistic ignorance. And even the large generalisations of Science are constantly found to apply to the truth of physical Nature formulas already discovered by the Indian sages in their original, their largest meaning the deeper truth of the spirit."

SRI AUROBINDO ON THE GITA

It was inevitable that the Gita should find an important place in a system of thought and spiritual practice as catholic and universal in spirit and application as Sri Aurobindo's. To Sri Aurobindo the Gita marks a crucial turn in the history of the development of Indian philosophy and religion. For, it takes up the diverse traditions and lines of thinking that had developed in the· post-Upanishadic age following the eclipse of the ancient Vedic Spirit and attempts a living synthesis of all the elements into one broad many-sided system assimilating into itself the fundamental truths of the Vedic and Upanishadic wisdom, harmonising their various strains and formulating them into forms and terms more suited to the mind of a later age.

Thus the Gita rescues the Vedic conception of sacrifice from the overgrowth of ritualism and hedonism that had succeeded in effectively covering the visage of the truth of *yajña*. It separates the basic truth of sacrifice from the restricted form it had come to acquire and presents it in its cosmic setting with bearings on each individual life. The Gita describes how sacrifice, self-giving, was the central lever on which the creator has set the machinery of the universe into operation, how life is governed by the principle of sacrifice at every level of creation. Man is called upon to recognise this truth of inner sacrifice as the key to his larger development and enjoined to train his faculties of body, life and mind and heart in the yoga of self-consecration, *yajña*, to the Divine, the Divine in himself, the Divine in All, the Divine in Nature, thereby forging a solidarity with the whole of creation and embracing the Divine Manifestation in a scheme of progressive self-enlargement and self-transcendence.

The Gita rights the balance of relation between man and the universe, between the individual and collectivity that had come to be tilted in the ascetic extremes of the period following the era of the earlier Upanishads. The emphasis had been shifted to the salvation of the individual in total disregard of the world which was looked upon as a field of ignorance and falsehood to be discarded. The Gita underlines the inter-relation of man and the environment in which he lives and thrives and calls upon the seeker of God to pursue his quest simultaneously on both the levels — individual and collective — through disinterested works, equality of soul and universality of outlook, and exert himself, even after self-liberation, for the world, *lokasaṁgraha*. In asking the seeker to pour his purified, and later his liberated, energies on the world, the Gita links up the Kingdom of the Spirit with the field of strife on Earth and opens a wide way for the upliftment of the latter towards the heights of Freedom and Harmony.

Another distinct contribution of far-reaching significance, points out Sri Aurobindo, is the resolution of the dichotomy of the Mutable, *kṣara*, and the Immutable, *akṣara*, Brahmans posed by the philosophies of different scholars, each claiming higher status to its own position. The Gita finds the reconciliation in its concept of Purushottama, the Transcendent Person of whom the personal and the impersonal are two poises, two aspects, in the creative Movement. Each derives its full value from the other and both find their intrinsic and completing truth in the Transcendent. The Purushottama presiding over the unmanifest and manifest in his absoluteness is the last word in this synthesis of apparent opposites in the creation.

The Doctrine of Purushottama opens the door of reconciliation to yet another set of oppositions, e.g. Knowledge, *jnāna*, Devotion, *bhakti*, Works, *karma*, in the field of spiritual effort. For by its emphasis on devotion, love for the supreme Lord culminating in utter *surrender* to the Divine, the Gita finds the meeting ground of common fulfilment among different lines of yoga. True Knowledge of the Divine melts in Love for the Divine; intense self-consecration through works flows into an adoration of Love for the Lord; full Love yields complete Knowledge of the Beloved, it pours itself into a delighted offering of Works to the Master of Love.

In his monumental work, *Essays on the Gita*, Sri Aurobindo expounds in modern terms many ancient spiritual concepts of importance cryptically mentioned in the Gita, e.g. *avatāra*, *vibhūti*, the truth of *svabhāva* and *svadharma*, self-being and self-law, the relativity of human standards, the overriding claims of the Divine Truth on man, etc. etc.

To conclude with Sri Aurobindo's words:

"The language of the Gita, the structure of thought, the combination and balancing of ideas belong neither to the temper of a sectarian teacher nor to the spirit of a vigorous analytical dialectics cutting off one angle of the truth to exclude all the others; but rather there is a wide, undulating, encircling movement of ideas which is the manifestation of a vast synthetic mind and rich synthetic experience. It does not cleave asunder, but reconciles and unifies.

"The Gita starts from the Vedantic synthesis and upon the basis of its essential ideas builds another harmony of the three great means and powers, Love, Knowledge and Works, through which the soul of man can directly approach and cast itself into the Eternal.

"The last, the closing supreme word of the Gita expressing the highest mystery is spoken in two brief, direct and simple *slokas* and these are left without further comment or enlargement to sink into the mind and reveal their own fullness of meaning in the soul's experience. For it is alone this inner incessantly extending experience that can make evident the infinite ideal of meaning with which are for ever pregnant these words in themselves apparently so slight and simple. Thus runs the secret of secrets, the highest most direct message of the Ishwara: "Become my-minded, my lover and adorer, a sacrificer to Me, bow thyself to Me, to Me thou shalt come, this is my pledge and promise to thee, for dear art thou to Me. Abandon all dharmas and take refuge in Me alone. I will deliver thee from all sin and evil, do not grieve."

SRI AUROBINDO ON THE TANTRA

The Tantra recovers its original purity and wide spiritual coverage in the integral approach of Sri Aurobindo. To him the Tantra is a part of the bequest of the ancient wisdom of the Veda. We have observed earlier how the Upanishads take up the Knowledge content of the older tradition and go on to develop it in a manner suited to the mind of a later day. The Tantra may be similarly said to continue and develop the esoteric part of the sadhana, the practice of inner culture and growth of the multiple being of man. Indeed, the Brahmanas took care of the outer ritual almost exclusively and erected quite a system out of it. But the methods of communication with the higher powers, the promotion of the community of interests among Man, Nature and God, which formed part of the more occult tradition were taken up and combined in the line of the Agamas, popularly known as the Tantras.

Sri Aurobindo appreciates the all-sided approach of the Tantra to the problem of man. It embraces the whole of man in its scheme; it does not make a radical division between his outer life and inner, lower and higher. It takes him in his totality and aims to give the fullest value to all the elements in his life, uplifting all the members of his being to participate in the divine joy of creation.

In this system there are two ends of the yoga-sadhana that are to be tapped. There is first a concentrated potential in the human system spread underneath

the surface. Only a fraction of it is normally active in
the life of man. This potential power is there latent
on all the planes of the being and the Science of Tantra
has located its points of concentration in certain regions of the body and called them chakras or involu-
tions. Through yogic processes such as pranayama,
japa etc. or by spiritual means like the touch or impact of the Guru or some Divine Grace, this Śakti —
Kundalini as it is termed — is awakened and drawn
upwards through chakra after chakra, the different locii
at different levels of the being and led to reach its
summit in the crown of the head where it meets its
Divine Lord.

The other end of the lever is the Higher Shakti, the
Divine Puissance, to which one surrenders oneself and
invokes for the liberating and fulfilling action. There
is a recognition that the main burden of the task is
borne by the Divine Power, the Mahashakti, the
Supreme Mother of the Universe. The individual shakti
is only one current of that ocean and in the conflu-
ence of the two the purpose is achieved.

The purpose, it must be noted, is not mukti, liberation alone. It includes bhukti, enjoyment of the Delight
of Life. The Divine creates the universe for the Bliss
of manifestation and the complete individual takes his
due share, participates in the cosmic Enjoyment as a
channel of the supreme Enjoyer. And Life excludes nothing. All elements, all movements have their due part
to play; according to his competence, adhikāra, the individual takes to the means appropriate to his nature.

To sum up in the words of Sri Aurobindo:

"Tantric discipline is in its nature a synthesis. It has seized on the large universal truth that there are two poles of being whose essential unity is the secret of existence, Brahman and Shakti, Spirit and Nature, and that Nature is power of the spirit or rather is spirit as power. To raise nature in man into manifest power of spirit is its method and it is the whole nature that it gathers up for the spiritual conversion. It includes in its system of instrumentation the forceful Hathayogic process and especially the opening up of the nervous centres and the passage through them of the awakened Shakti on her way to her union with the Brahman, the subtler stress of the Rajayogic purification, meditation and concentration, the leverage of will-force, the motive power of devotion, the key of knowledge. But it does not stop short with an effective assembling of the different powers of these specific Yogas. In two directions it enlarges by its synthetic turn the province of the Yogic method. First, it lays its hand firmly on many of the main springs of the human quality, desire, action and it subjects them to an intensive discipline with the soul's mastery of its motives as first aim and their elevation to a diviner spiritual level as its final utility. Again it includes in its objects of Yoga not only liberation, which is the one all-mastering preoccupation of the specific systems, but a cosmic enjoyment of the power of the Spirit, which the others may take incidentally on the way, in part, casually, but

3

avoid making a motive or object. It is a bolder and larger system."

No wonder some of the main principles of this Science of Tantra enter into the scheme of Sri Aurobindo's Integral Yoga. To quote from him again:

"The ascent of the consciousness through the centres and other Tantric knowledge are there behind the process of transformation to which so much importance is given by me; also the truth that nothing can be done except through the force of the Mother."

Further,

"The process of the Kundalini awakened rising through the centres as also the purification of the centres is a Tantric knowledge. In our yoga there is no willed process of the purification and opening of the centres, no raising up of the Kundalini by a set process either. Another method is used, but still there is the ascent of the consciousness from and through the different levels to join the higher consciousness above; there is the opening of the centres and of the planes (mental, vital, physical) which these centres command; there is also the descent which is the main key of the spiritual transformation. Therefore, there is a Tantric knowledge behind the process of transformation in this yoga."

SRI AUROBINDO ON INDIAN CULTURE

In a series of articles in the ARYA which began with a review article on the *Renaissance in India* by Dr. James Cousins, and another series* provoked by an insensate attack on Indian culture by William Archer, Sri Aurobindo analyses the basis and the motivating spirit of Indian culture.

The culture of a people is the way of life, thought and action developed by them to express certain values that have a special appeal to their collective Soul. Thus ancient Greece cherished the ideals of Beauty of form and elegance of mind and their culture and civilisation was characterised by a seeking for these truths. Similarly the Roman life was governed by a spirit of organisation, of Law and Order, that of Hebrews by an ethical strain, of the Japanese by love of Art. The dominant note of the Indian life-effort, Sri Aurobindo points out, has been the spiritual.

To say that the character of Indian culture is spiritual does not mean that it is life-shunning and other-worldly. Its spirituality, on the contrary, is all-embracing. The whole of life is invested with a deep significance of the Spirit. In this perspective, all existences, all movements in the universe are part of a vast manifesting Spirit. There is a Divine Reality behind and above all that lives and moves, originating all, governing all, leading all. Life is an effort to express this

* In three sequences entitled, *Is India Civilised? A Rationalistic Critic on Indian Culture* and *A Defence of Indian Culture.*

Divine Reality, its Consciousness in a growing manner. The early dawns of the Veda see an open avowal of this perception and Faith in the divine purpose of man's life-journey. All is One in this basic Consciousness — all worlds, their inhabitants, all powers and beings are one in the one Divine. Behind all the apparent diversity there is this Oneness. The aim of life is to realise this consciousness of Divinity and manifest it in the diverse fields of activity.

This is the central motive of Indian life from the beginning. And the best periods in the growth and efflorescence of the Indian civilisation has been those in which the people have kept close to this Ideal and vision. Periods of decline have been precisely those when this inspiration has been relegated to the background and lesser attractions have occupied the people.

It is said by Western critics that the religious and spiritual turn of the Indian people has been the cause of their material downfall. Exposing the absurdity of this charge, Sri Aurobindo points out how this very turn in the character of the Indian race has raised the value of life in all its gradations, in all its movements and invested it with a profound meaning. The whole of life is looked upon as a journey from Ignorance to Knowledge, from limitation and incapacity to Power and Strength, from pain and suffering to Joy and Bliss. All the branches of life-activity are geared to this purpose — Art, Literature, Science, Philosophy, Polity — and no gulf is left unbridged between Earth and Heaven. Matter is regarded as the robe of the Spirit and the Spirit as the soul of Matter. The celebrated sixty-four arts of Indian knowledge interpret the one in terms of the other and link them both in the consciousness of man. *Sarvam khalu idam brahma,* All this is verily Brahman; *ayamātmā brahma,* this self is Brahman: *tat twamasi,* That thou art; these are the ringing truths reverberating in the Indian consciousness down the ages.

A fundamental tenet of faith in this approach is the truth of Karma. Here again, belief in Karma has not made the people pessimistic and prone to fatalism as the critics think. The perception that there is a law of action and reaction in life makes man awake to his responsibility in determining his future. He has it in his hands to shape his destiny. The corollary of the truth of Rebirth gives an enlarged perspective of the goal of life. The knowledge that this one brief tenure of life on earth is not all and that one has an eternity of time in which to grow and perfect oneself in the image of God gives a security and poise to the awakened individual that lifts him out of the fevered stampede of hurrying life.

If the Indian mind believes in Fate, a cosmic Will that effectuates itself regardless of individual conveniences, it also knows that this will operates through so many constituent individual wills and that there is a Divine Grace transcending all determinisms — individual and universal — a grace which can be invoked by a soul-movement. All religions, all philosophies in India recognise the omnipotent character of this Power of

Divine Grace.

Thus man is regarded as a conscious participant in the manifestation of the Divine that is this universe, a being who can determine the direction and the pace of his journey towards the eventual goal of divine perfection and freedom. Even the Gods are his helpers, the earth is the chosen field for this progression of man. This is the central Idea in the Indian outlook and the culture based upon it.

To sum up in the words of Sri Aurobindo:

"Spirituality is indeed the master-key of the Indian mind; the sense of the infinite is native to it. India saw from the beginning — and, even in her ages of reason and her age of increasing ignorance, she never lost hold of the insight — that life cannot be rightly seen in the sole light, cannot be perfectly lived in the sole power of its externalities. She was alive to the greatness of material laws and forces; she had a keen eye for the importance of the physical sciences; she knew how to organise the arts of ordinary life. But she saw that the physical does not get its full sense until it stands in right relation to the supra-physical; she saw that the complexity of the universe could not be explained in the present terms of man or seen by his superficial sight, that there were other powers behind, other powers within man himself of which he is normally unaware, that he is conscious only of a small part of himself, that the invisible always surrounds the visible, the suprasensible the sensible, even as infinity always surrounds the finite.

"She saw too that man has the power of exceeding himself, of becoming himself more entirely and profoundly than he is, truths which have only recently begun to be seen in Europe and seem even now too great for its common intelligence. She saw the myriad gods beyond man, God beyond the gods, and beyond God his own ineffable eternity: she saw that there were ranges of mind beyond our present mind and above these she saw the splendours of the spirit. Then with that calm audacity of her intution which knew no fear or littleness and shrank from no act whether of spiritual or intellectual, ethical or vital courage, she declared that there was none of these things which man could not attain if he trained his will and knowledge; he could conquer these ranges of mind, become the spirit, become a god, become one with God, become the ineffable Brahman. And with the logical practicality and sense of science and organised method which distinguished her mentality, she set forth immediately to find out the way. Hence from long ages of this insight and practice there was ingrained in her spirituality, her powerful psychic tendency, her great yearning to grapple with the infinite and possess it, her ineradicable religious sense, her idealism, her Yoga, the constant turn of her art and her philosophy.

"But this was not and could not be her whole mentality, her entire spirit; spirituality itself does not flourish on earth in the void, even as our mountain-tops do not rise like that of an enchantment of dream

out of the clouds without a base. When we look at
the past of India, what strikes us next is her stupendous vitality, her inexhaustible power of life and joy
of life, her almost unimaginably prolific creativeness.
For three thousand years at least — it is indeed much
longer — she has been creating abundantly and incessantly, lavishly, with an inexhaustible many-sidedness,
republics and kingdoms and empires, philosophies and
cosmogonies and sciences and creeds and arts and
poems and all kinds of monuments, palaces and temples
and public works, communities and societies and religious orders, laws and codes and rituals, physical
sciences, psychic sciences, systems of Yoga, systems of
politics and administration, arts spiritual, arts worldly,
trades, industries, fine crafts — the list is endless and
in each item there is almost a plethora of activity. She
creates and creates and is not satisfied and is not
tired; she will not have an end of it, seems hardly to
need a space for rest, a time for inertia and lying
fallow. She expands too outside her borders; her ships
cross the ocean and the fine superfluity of her wealth
brims over to Judea and Egypt and Rome; her colo-
nies spread her arts and epics and creeds in the Archi-
pelago; her traces are found in sands of Mesopotamia;
her religions conquer China and Japan and spread
westward as far as Palestine and Alexandria, and the
figures of the Upanishads and the sayings of the Bud-
dhists are re-echoed on the lips of Christ. Everywhere,
as on her soil, so in her works there is the teeming of
a super-abundant energy of life."

And what of the future?

"The spiritual motive will be in the future of India, as in her past, the real originative and dominating strain. By spirituality we do not mean a remote metaphysical mind or the tendency to dream rather than to act. That was not the great India of old in her splendid days of vigour, — whatever certain European critics or interpreters of her culture may say, — and it will not be the India of the future. Metaphysical thinking will always no doubt be a strong element in her mentality, and it is to be hoped that she will never lose her great, her sovereign powers in that direction; but Indian metaphysics is as far removed from the brilliant or the profound idea spinning of the French or the German mind as from the broad intellectual generalising on the basis of the facts of physical science which for some time did duty for philosophy in modern Europe. It has always been in its essential parts an intellectual approach to spiritual realisation. Though in later time it led too much away from life, yet that was not its original character whether in its early Vedantic intuitional forms or in those later developments of it, such as the Gita, which belong to the period of its most vigorous intellectual originality and creation. Buddhism itself, the philosophy which first really threw doubt on the value of life, did so only in its intellectual tendency; in its dynamic parts, by its ethical system and spiritual method, it gave a new set of values, a severe vigour, yet a gentler idealism to human living and was therefore powerfully creative both in the arts which interpret life and in society and politics. To realise intimately truth of spirit and to quicken and to remould life by it is the native tendency of the Indian mind, and to that it must always return in all its periods of health, greatness and vigour."

SRI AUROBINDO ON SOCIAL DEVELOPMENT

It is not the individual man alone who undergoes spiritual evolution. The society in which he lives is also evolving in the same direction. And that is inevitable because both — the individual and the collectivity — are self-formulations of one Divine Reality with the same purpose — the expression of the manifesting Spirit.

Sri Aurobindo perceives in the growth of the society an ordered, progressive evolution. As in the case of the individual, the rudiments of the soul gradually take shape and a collective soul gets formed and develops in the direction of a spiritual fulfilment. This progression may be studied in three or four well-marked steps of growth.

As a rule a strong religious and symbolic spirit governs the mind of man in the early stages of society. Instinctively man feels and recognises some higher Powers at work in Nature and he submits himself to their care. Everything in life symbolises to him something other than, and greater than the appearance. His life is crowded with the influences and activities of Powers and Beings greater than himself and he forges a relation between himself and the Powers or Gods through ritual, prayer, adoration and the like. Such are the early societies of the Vedic Aryans, the Mystics of Greece, Egypt etc. This is the first, the *Symbolic Age*.

This live organism of society, however, tends to fix

itself into an organisation. Gradually there emerges a
typal order with certain sections performing certain
duties and the society falls into distinct constituent types.
The living ritual of religion, dynamic movement of the
inner spirit, the spontaneously growing and self-adjusting
norms of the society begin to petrify into fixed conven-
tions and ill-understood customs. The climax of this
Typal and Conventional Age comes when the society is
over-burdened by this mechanical apparatus of Law and
Custom and the individual questions and revolts.

This ushers in the third age, the *Age of Individualism
and Reason.* Everything is challenged, the human mind
armed with reason questions every custom and every
faith. Man asserts his right to think and chalk out for
himself his path of progress. The general result of this
double movement of destruction and freedom is to pull
down the old structure of time-worn Custom and Law,
to break down many walls of superstition and dogma
that bar the route to progress. Reason probes everywhere, plumbs into the depths of existence, in order to
find the basic truth of life. Now it seems to have found
it in physical Matter, now in life-energy, now in a mental substance. It cannot rest anywhere because fresh evidence constantly turns up exposing the inadequacy of its
formed conclusions and pointing to other possibilities.
The thinker moves from materialism to vitalism and
thence to mentalism; when all these are found insuffi-
cient to guide towards an effective government and
direction of life, he steps into the subjective era; he
is faced with testimonies of the existence of a belt of

existence behind the veil of the surface exterior — the subliminal which is the seat of the many para-psychological and psychical phenomena that exceed the range of mental reason. The present age of humanity is this *Subjective Age*; man confesses to the existence of a supra-rational range of life and awakens to faculties within himself that correspond to the realities of this order of life — the faculties of telepathy, pre-sight, intuition, inspiration, etc.

The culmination of this subjective movement is the entry into the fourth, the *Spiritual Age* in which all routes lead to the truth of the Soul. Man discovers his true centre of existence in the soul, a divine entity at the core of his being and equally a pervading Spirit in the universe. He further realises that at this soul-level all existence is One. The self of the individual, *atman*, and the Self of the universe, *brahman*, are the same. Once this truth is perceived and realised there is an irresistible movement towards Harmony, Commonalty and Unity. The Truth of the manifesting Spirit begins to organise itself in the collectivity of the Human Race.

To quote from Sri Aurobindo: "having set out with a symbolic age, an age in which man felt a great Reality behind all life which he sought through symbols, it (mind of man) will reach an age in which it will begin to live in that Reality, not through the symbol, not by the power of the type or of the convention or of the individual reason and intellectual will, but in our own highest nature which will be the nature of

that Reality fulfilled in the conditions — not necssarily
the same as now — of terrestrial existence. This is what
the religions have seen with a more or less adequate
intuition, but most often as in a glass darkly, that
which they called the kingdom of God on earth, —
his kingdom within in men's spirit and therefore, for
the one is the material result of the effectivity of the
other, his kingdom without in the life of the peoples."

SRI AUROBINDO ON HUMAN
UNITY

The problem of collectivity does not cease with the establishment of a harmonious relation between the individual and the collective society. What about the relations between the various societies among themselves and also between the collectivities and the still larger collectivity of humanity? Here too Sri Aurobindo proceeds on the spiritual truth of manifestation: the One basing and containing the Many, Diversity in Unity.

He traces the growth of man in collectivity from the very beginning of aggregate development. For apparent reasons of security and survival — though in truth under a deeper impulsion of Nature in her drive towards unity from primal fragmentation — man collects around himself his family members and forms the first unit. The family develops into the commune. Then comes the tribe or the clan. Each unit leads to a bigger unit. Cities, principalities, petty kingdoms follow in progression till the nation-unit is arrived at.

The Nation is the strongest collective unit so far devised by Nature to give shape to the group-life and group-soul of a people who develop a common culture, common ideals and common ways of living. Such people tend to gather and organise themselves into a distinct nation with a stamp of its own.

But, Sri Aurobindo points out, the nation is only the intermediate unity. Each nation confronting other nations, defensively or even offensively, is certainly not the last word in the collective evolution of humanity. Nature is striving to form a yet larger aggregation without hurting the life impulses and soul-aspirations of the peoples constituting the nations. History records many and varied attempts in this direction: empires, commonwealths, federations, confederacies and the like. The goal Nature aims at is to found a large unit of family of Nation in which each constituting unit is a thriving member drawing upon the commonalty for its progress but at the same time freely contributing its share to the general well-being of the whole.

Sri Aurobindo describes this process in history in detail and confidently foresees the eventual establishment of One World comity of nations in which all nations shall have equal rights, regardless of their size or development, though each may have a natural influence corresponding to its resources. He regards the founding of the League of Nations as the first notable step on the political plane in this direction. It failed but its very failure has contributed to the rise of a better and more effective worldbody in the United Nations Organisation. Here too the inherent defects in its structure and modes of functioning are likely to defeat its purpose and unless they are remedied and the organisation re-formed in time, it also is likely to go the way of its predecessor and a third attempt will have to be undertaken if humanity is to survive. To use an old phrase, the UNO has either to be mended or ended to make way for another Organisation more in tune with the collective aspirations

of the peoples and capable of building up a new era
of oneness and peace.

Sri Aurobindo warns, however, that all fresh efforts
to erect organisations to achieve world peace, world
unity etc. can only succeed in forming outer structures.
They are to be made alive and turned into dynamic
instruments for progress by breathing into them the
living spirit of harmony and peace and oneness by the
men and women who represent humanity in evolution.
This underlines the need for the realisation of the truth
of unity and harmony on the psychological and soul
level on the part of the leaders of thought and life in
the collective movement of humanity.

Sri Aurobindo originally wrote this series under the
title "*Ideal of Human Unity*" between the years 1915-
1918, in the pages of the ARYA. When he turned to
them again three decades later — 1949 — to see if any
revision was called for in the light of subsequent developments on the world-scene, there was no need to
change any of the main conclusions. They were found to
have been largely confirmed and fresh departures
already anticipated. Writing a Postscript he envisaged
an era of co-existence between the two blocks of the
communist and non-comunist Ideologies. He foresaw the
emergence of China as a militant Power and warned:

"In Asia a more perilous situation has arisen, stand-
ing sharply across the way to any possibility of a continental unity of the peoples of this part of the world
in the emergence of a communist China. This creates

4

a gigantic block which could easily englobe the whole of Northern Asia in a combination between two enormous communist powers, Russia and China and would overshadow with a threat of absorption South-Western Asia and Tibet and might be pushed to overrun all up to the whole frontier of India menacing her security and that of Western Asia with the possibility of an invasion and an overrunning and subjection by penetration or even by overwhelming military force to an unwanted ideology, political and social institutions and dominance of this militant mass of Communism whose push might easily prove irresistible."

What of the world's future?

"The ultimate result must be the formation of a World-State and the most desirable form of it would be a federation of free nationalities in which all subjection or forced inequality and subordination of one to another would have disappeared and, though some might preserve a greater natural influence, all would have an equal status. A confederacy would give the greatest freedom to the nations constituting the World-State, but this might give too much room for fissiparous or centrifugal tendencies to operate: a federal order would then be most desirable. All else would be determined by the course of events and by general agreement or the shape given by the ideas and neccessities that may grow up in future. A world union of this kind would have the greatest chances of long survival or permanent existence."

SRI AUROBINDO'S EPIC *SAVITRI*

A substantial part of Sri Aurobindo's writings is poetry and on poetry. To Sri Aurobindo poetry, like all art, is an interpreter of the Reality, whether finite or infinite. It is not a decorative element in life. True poetry communicates an experience, a message, a vision of truth. It embodies something that is lived by the soul and seeks to communicate it. It follows that the word to convey this truth must carry its characteristic vibration. It must answer to the quality of the message that seeks expression. Poetry is thus a living vehicle of truth-experience. It not only records the experience but is potent enough to communicate it to the reader or hearer. This in fact was the nature of the poetry of the ancient Vedic Rishis or the seers of the Upanishad. The Mantra was the inevitable word that came vibrating out of their spiritual depths and took shape in the mind. Sri Aurobindo perceives that with the turn of the Soul of humanity towards the Truth of the Spirit, poetry is on its way to assume its rightful function and he expounds the direction in which world-poetry is fast developing. He himself has written a great body of poetry — and prose poetry — illustrating this movement towards a living expression of mystic truth. The *tour de force* in this field is his work *Savitri: A Legend and a Symbol* — the longest epic in the English language — running into twenty-three thousand lines and more.

Sri Aurobindo draws upon the well-known story of

Savitri-Satyavan from the Vanaparva of the Mahabharata but in his hands it ceases to be a mere didactic narrative extolling the virtues of wifely devotion. As a Legend and a Symbol it is at once the spiritual history of the world and the epic of man in his struggle from Darkness, Falsehood and Death to Light, Truth and Immortality.

Sri Aurobindo gives full value to the significance of the names used by the seers of old and develops his theme following the suggestions thrown out by them. King Asvapati is the Lord of Life (*aśva* in the ancient thought represents Life-energy), the representative man who has arrived at the acme of human evolution and seeks to break out of the limitations imposed by Nature upon Man. For this purpose he enters into a journey of exploration of his own inner being and then upwards into the spiritual heights of Existence. He becomes the Pilgrim of the Spirit and climbs along the stair of the Planes of Creation, comes face to face with different formulations of the creative Consciousness and Power, understands in these terms much of the mystery of life on earth, and finally arrives at the summit where the Glory of the Divine Being is fully manifest. He aspires to establish this Truth, Light and Bliss on Earth in the conditions of Ignorance, obscurity and suffering and for that purpose he entreats the Divine Mother of All to come down and manifest the Divine Verities on Earth. The Divine Mother promises that an emanation of Her Grace will be born as his daughter to achieve this object:

O strong forerunner, I have heard thy cry.
One shall descend and break the iron Law,
Change Nature's doom by the lone Spirit's power.
A limitless Mind that can contain the world,
A sweet and violent heart of ardent calms
Moved by the passions of the gods shall come.
All mights and greatness shall join in her;
Beauty shall walk celestial on the earth,
Delight shall sleep in the cloud-net of her hair
And in her body as on his homing tree
Immortal Love shall beat his glorious wings.
A music of griefless things shall weave her charm;
The harps of the Perfect shall attune her voice,
The streams of Heaven shall murmur in her laugh,
Her lips shall be the honeycombs of God,
Her limbs his golden jars of ecstasy,
Her breasts the rapture-flowers of Paradise.
She shall bear Wisdom in her voiceless bosom,
Strength shall be with her like a conqueror's sword
And from her eyes the Eternal's bliss shall gaze.
A seed shall be sown in Death's tremendous hour,
A branch of heaven transplant to human soil;
Nature shall overleap her mortal step;
Fate shall be changed by an unchanging will.

In due time, an effulgent daughter is born and is appropriately named *Savitri*, issued from Savitr, the Sun of Truth. She grows up in the palace of King Asvapati and at a pregnant moment her father asks her to go forth in the country and choose her life-companion.

And Savitri chooses *Satyavan* (he who has the Truth) in a forest where his father *Dyumatsena* (leader of the hosts of light) lives in exile. This captain of light is blinded and banished from his rightful possessions.* However, it turns out that Satyavan is fated to die within a year and her parents advise her to make another choice, which she refuses to do. Sage Narada who reveals this decree of Fate applauds her decision and wishes her godspeed in her resolve to stake all for the sake of Satyavan, the Man of Truth. He tells the queen-mother:

She only can save herself and save the world.
O queen, stand back from that stupendous scene,
Come not between her and her hour of Fate.
Her hour must come and none can intervene:
Think not to turn her from her heaven-sent task,
Strive not to save her from her own high will.
Thou hast no place in that tremendous strife;
Their love and longing are not arbiters there,
Leave the world's fate and her to God's sole guard.
Even if he seems to leave her to her lone strength,
Even though all falters and falls and sees an end
And the heart fails and only are death and night,
God-given her strength can battle against doom
Even on a brink where Death alone seems close
And no human strength can hinder or can help.

* The imagery is plain enough. Though he is at the head of the evolutionary army of Light, Man blinded by Ignorance, forfeits his Kingdom.

Think not to intercede with the hidden Will,
Intrude not twixt her spirit and its force
But leave her to her mighty self and Fate.

The fateful day dawns, Satyavan is claimed by the
Great Woodsman and an epic encounter takes place
between Savitri who is conscious of her divinity and
Yama the God of Death. In a memorable debate all
the strategems of Deceit and Falsehood employed by
the Adversary are exposed and the Truth of Divine
Manifestation established. Death is forced to dissolve:

His body was eaten by light, his spirit devoured.
At last he knew defeat inevitable
And left crumbling the shape that he had worn,
Abandoning hope to make man's soul his prey
And force to be mortal the immortal spirit.
Afar he fled shunning her dreaded touch
And refuge took in the retreating Night.
In the dream twilight of that symbol world
The dire universal Shadow disappeared
Vanishing into the Void from which it came.

and Immortality for Man is won.

It is a Vast Canvas on which the entire gamut of
thought, emotion, passion and action of men and gods,
titans and angels, forces and beings is portrayed. The
various worlds and their organisations are described
vividly. Philosophies, religions, sciences find their
echoes here. Age-old antagonists like Good and Evil,
Truth and Falsehood, Light and Darkness, fight out

their battles in a spectacular manner. The old order crumbles and the Dawn of the New Age approaches:

Night, splendid with the moon dreaming in heaven
In silver peace, possessed her luminous reign.
She brooded through her stillness on a thought
Deep-guarded by her mystic folds of light,
And in her bosom nursed a greater dawn.

SRI AUROBINDO LITERATURE

On the occasion of the hundredth Birthday Anniversary of Sri Aurobindo on August 15, 1972, a definitive edition of all his published works is under issue. It covers 30 large Volumes of 500 pages each, and the last Volume is expected to be out well in time. The Centenary Edition is being brought out by Sri Aurobindo Ashram at Pondicherry and has created a world-wide interest. It will be useful to know the main subjects on which Sri Aurobindo has written. Sri Aurobindo literature consists, indeed, of his own writings spread over more than 50 years of his historic career. By way of elucidation and application, it necessarily includes the authentic writings of the Mother who has been his collaborator in the great endeavour of a New Life initiated by him. It also includes the growing number of books written by his disciples in the course of their life-long studies of the Master's Teachings.

The number of subjects on which Sri Aurobindo has written is incredibly large. And that is as it should be. For his vision embraces the whole of life and he believes in applying the God-Light he has gained to every nook and corner of man's existence. However, we shall begin with his *magnus opus* "The Life Divine" in which he presents the metaphysics of his conception and the Ideal of Divine Life for man.

The Life Divine

In this work Sri Aurobindo examines the two leading movements of human thought, the Materialist Denial (of God) and the Refusal of the Ascetic (to accept the world), and points out the services and the disservices rendered by them to the cause of human progress. He propounds his theory of Creation and the nature of the world-movement, based upon the perception of the seers of the Veda and the Upanishads; examines the connotation of Maya in the light of the older Wisdom and traces the course taken by the earth-evolution from the primal beginnings in the inconscient Waters of the Rig Veda through the stages of Matter (*anna*), Life (*prāṇa*), Mind (*manas*) and presently emerging into the belt of a spiritual consciousness pointing to a Gnosis termed the *ṛta cit* in the Veda. He discusses in detail how this Creation represents the projection of the Supreme Reality of *saccidānanda*, the causes for the appearance of Ignorance and Evil in the course of this Movement and the way of ascent from Darkness to Light, from Death to Immortality. The concepts of Brahman, Purusha, Ishwara and Maya, Prakriti, Shakti are expounded at length. So too the origins and the boundaries of the Ignorance, the seven ways of Knowledge, the philosophy of Rebirth, the order of the Worlds and the evolution of the spiritual man. In the last chapter, Sri Aurobindo visualises the lines on which a Gnostic community, the forerunner of a new race with a new consciousness, is likely to come into being and grow. He draws attention to confirmatory evidence in the developments of the world pointing to the emergence of the Superman endowed with the faculty of Truth-Intelligence and Truth-Power. In sum, this great work justifies God's labour in this universe and predicts confidently the kingdom of God on earth in the forseeable future, the *satya yuga*.

This book running into a thousand pages and more of classic prose in English, ringing celestial music in the ears of the reader reaches profound heights of thought, and the student may need to be helped at certain curves of the argument. For this purpose Chandrasekharan's *A Brief Study of the Life Divine*, Purani's *Lectures* (on L. D.), Bannerji's *Short Treatise* (on L. D.) are helpful. S. K. Maitra's *Meeting of East and West in Sri Aurobindo's Philosophy* is a comparative study.

The Life Divine has been translated into several languages: French, Hindi, Bengali, Marathi, Chinese. Translations are under way in Kannada, Gujarati and Italian.

THE SYNTHESIS OF YOGA

If *The Life Divine* is the *jnanapada*, the Knowledge-content of this *darshana*, *The Synthesis of Yoga* is the *yogapada*, the Science to translate the theory into practice. To Sri Aurobindo's yoga, inner discipline of askesis, is the sole means of achieving the object of Divine Life. For this purpose he expounds the main principle of yoga which is to tap and develop any one power of the human system so as to arrive at its fruition in its divine term. He traces the specialised applications of this principle to the powers of human will, intellect, emotions. He examines the theory and practice of the Yoga of Works, the Yoga of Knowledge, the Yoga of Love as they have been handed down the ages; he also discusses the rationale of Hatha Yoga, Raja Yoga, Samadhi and allied yogic practices. After evaluating their contribution to the spiritual development of man and noting their limitations when pursued exclusively, he develops his own Yoga of Self-Perfection into which the main elements of all these yogas enter in some form or other, at some stage or other. This yoga, the integral or *pūrṇayoga* as it is called, aims at the fusion of the individual, the cosmic and the transcendental spiritual realisation in man, leaving nothing of his existence unclaimed, transforming everything of him into a divine perfection.

Sri Aurobindo is not content with laying down the science. He takes pains to guide the practicants on the routes he has chalked out. He answers in detail and in simple language the innumerable questions, problems posed by the disciples and other interested enquirers in the course of their study and practice. These answers of invaluable import have been collected together in the three Volumes of *Letters on Yoga*. Thousands of letters have been collected, edited, classified under suitable heads: Foundations, Difficulties, Requirements, Dreams and Experiences, Sex, Food, Sleep, Transformation of Physical Nature, Vital Nature, Mental Nature, the Emotions, the Psychic Being and its role in the liberation, Attitude to Life, Works as a means and a field for spiritual progress, Mental Doubt and the way to meet it, Death, After-death passage, process of Rebirth, Out-of-the-body experiences and many other topics of relevance to the sadhaka.

Equal in importance are the writings and conversations of the Mother who answers (over a period of fifty years) questions from children of ten up to adults of ninety on yoga, life and super-life. The light the Mother throws on the occult side of existence is authentic and clears a good deal of confusion and superstition prevalent regarding the subtler planes of the universe, the several personalities of man, the operation of Laws of Nature behind the veil. After reading the Mother's writings it is impossible to have fear or doubt. Next, there are helpful and expository writings by the disciples. Nolini Kanta Gupta's *Yoga of Sri Aurobindo* (eleven parts), Kapali Sastriar's *Lights on the Teachings,* Rishabhchand's *Integral Yoga of Sri Aurobindo*, Pandit's *Sadhana in Sri Aurobindo's Yoga, The Call and The Grace, Japa, Dhyana* and *All Life is Yoga* (six parts), are found particularly helpful.

Both the *Synthesis* and the *Letters* have been translated into Hindi, Marathi, French and Chinese. Translations are being done in parts in other languages.

It is often asked if Sri Aurobindo is a Vedantin or a Tantric. Well, he himself has said that he uses the method of the Vedanta to arrive at the goal of the Tantra. And the goal of the Tantra, as we know, is to possess the world as a creation of the Divine Consciousness for the enjoyment of the Divine Being realised in oneself. The whole of life is conceived as an outpouring of the Divine Puissance, Shakti which is formulated in the cosmos as the *Mahāśakti* and in the individual as the Kundalini. It is the Divine Shakti that creates; it is again the same Shakti that liberates. Consciousness, Power, Grace, all these are so many facets of one Divine Reality, conceived and experienced by the awakened human soul as the Divine Mother. This is a self-evident truth in the tradition of the Tantra and Sri Aurobindo makes of this truth the cornerstone of the edifice of his yoga. For this purpose, he has written that gem of a book, *The Mother*, which is both the Bible and the Gita in the Shastra of this New Yoga. In this little prose-poem, Sri Aurobindo delineates the manifestation of the Four major Cosmic Powers from the One Adya Shakti, Primal Power, e.g. Maheshwari, Mahakali, Mahalaxmi and Mahasaraswati, and in precise terms describes the part they play in the evolution of the world, individually in men and collectively in mankind. He lays down the conditions that man has to fulfil before he can be conscious of their divine working in his being and the role they play in his future evolution.

This book has been translated into Sanskrit and almost all Indian languages and in French, German, Chinese etc.

Sri Aurobindo also integrates in his system certain other principles of the Tantra, e.g. the existence of several centres of consciousness in the subtle body of man, the function of worship, mantra, self-surrender to the Divine Power for effecting the release and transformation. He has shown how the Tantric tradition follows the Vedic in a natural manner. If the Upanishads represents the knowledge-element of the Vedic past, the Mimamsa the ritual content, the Tantra formulates and continues the esoteric side of the Vedic heritage. Kapali Sastriar proves in his *Sidelights on the Tantra* the continuity in the two traditions, explains how the *yajna* developed into *yāga*, how even the very same mantras from the Veda are used on certain important occasions in the Tantra. His disciple Pandit has followed up this trend of thought with his *Lights on the Tantra, Kundalini Yoga, Studies in the Tantras and the Veda*, two series of *Gems from the Tantras* and his renderings of the *Kularnava Tantra*. Another disciple of Sastriar, S. Shankaranarayanan has written knowledgably on *Devī Māhātmyam* (in English and Tamil), *Śri Cakra* and *The Daśa Mahāvidyās*. He has examined the ancient concepts in these traditions in the light of modern thought and shown how they yield their full meaning and value when presented in the framework of Sri Aurobindo's Yoga and Philosophy, particularly as described in his Epic *Savitri*.

VEDA

It was natural that Sri Aurobindo should turn to the authentic Indian Scriptures of old to see what corroboration he could find for the synthesis he had already arrived at in the course of his tapasya. He was agreeably surprised to find the Rig Veda bear testimony to a line of positive spiritual effort made by the ancients in the early dawns of the Indian civilisation. He went straight to the heart of that great Litany and found that the hymns recorded an ascent of the human soul towards the highest Godhead symbolised by the Vedic Sun. The Rishis emerge from these riks as mystics who are engaged in building the various gods in themselves, i.e. in manifesting the divine Powers for the full possession and fulfilment of life on earth. They have their own system of worlds and the gods presiding over them and their technique of actualising those states of existence in themselves. This, says Sri Aurobindo, is the central purpose, the kernel of the Veda, the *adhyatmic* content referred to by teachers like Yaska. He does not question that the Vedic treasury may and does contain coins of other denominations, but the spiritual is the most precious. He has embodied the results of his studies in the Veda in two series: *Secret of the Veda, Selected Hymns* (including Hymns to Agni).

Underlining this character of the yoga of the Vedic Rishis as a yoga of fulfilment and not of withdrawal from the world, Kapali Sastriar has written the *Sid-*

dhānjana, a commentary in Sanskrit on the first *aṣṭaka* of the Rig Veda, rik by rik, explaining and justifying the esoteric interpretations. His hundred-page introduction to the work has been already issued in English. A summary of it is to be found in his *Lights on the Veda* and *Further Lights on the Veda*. The whole of the *Siddhānjana* is currently being translated in English by Pandit and Shankaranarayanan. Pandit's studies, *Mystic approach to the Veda and the Upanishad*, *Aditi and other Deities in the Veda*, *Key to Vedic Symbolism* and Purani's *Studies in Vedic Interpretation* and *Vedic Glossary* throw helpful light on the subject. Nolini Gupta's *Madhuchhandamala* in Bengali has made a name for itself.

Sri Aurobindo's work on the Veda has been trans-lated in Hindi, Tamil, French and Chinese.

UPANISHADS

Sri Aurobindo discerns a clear variation in the tone and spirit of the older Upanishads and the later ones. Of these older texts he has commented in detail on the Isha and the Kena and shown how they tackle the problem of equating of this world with Brahman, life on earth with the bliss of the Transcendent, the body with the soul. That the universe is a willed self-projection of the Lord, the One who enters individually into the Many and that character of this creation is one of increasing manifestation of the Divine Truth

5

and the goal of man is to realise the Divine Consciousness in himself and radiate it in the life around, is the message of the Upanishad. He has translated the Isha, Kena, Taittiriya, Aitareya, Mundaka, Mandukya, Katha and the Svetasvatara Upanishads. In his essays on the *Philosophy of the Upanishads* and studies into the spirit of the Upanishads he expounds how the Upanishads are a body of one homogenous thought verified and verifiable in spiritual experience, how they are vehicles of illumination with purposive intervals of thought, enlarging continuations of the Vedic tradition and not — as Western scholars believe — revolts against the older tradition and guesses of thought of heterogenous minds.

Kapali Sastriar examines in his *Lights on the Upanishads,* certain important Vidyas, e.g. *prana vidya, sandilya vidya, vaishvanara vidya, madhu vidya* etc. in the light of this approach and shows how the Upanishads are manuals of sadhana. Pandit's *Upanishads: Gateways of Knowledge, Guide to the Upanishads, Essence of the Upanishads* and *Gleanings from the Upanishads* have been welcomed. Nolini Gupta's writings in his *Seers and Poets, Poets and Mystics* expound the symbolism in these ancient texts.

GITA

Of all the Indian Scriptures, the Bhagavad Gita may be said to have had the most profound effect upon the mind of Sri Aurobindo, especially in his pre-Pondicherry days. He himself refers to his frequent use of this work for purposes of his sadhana while in jail. And perhaps the largest number of references to Sanskrit Scriptures in his writings are to the Gita. Sri Aurobindo does not approach the Gita for support to any pre-conceived system of philosophy but enters with an open mind so as to grasp direct the message of the Lord. In his *Essays on the Gita* he draws attention to the synthetic character of the work harmonising the different spiritual traditions prevalent at that time and focusses special attention on the doctrine of Purushottama reconciling the *kshara* and the *akshara purushas*, the doctrine of selfless action promoting liberation through the very works which normally form the bondage. He highlights the divine call to resist evil in whatever form, to act according to the imperatives of the soul irrespective of the claims of the conflicting man-made *dharma*. To Sri Aurobindo the Gita is a spiritual manual whose dynamic import is as relevant today as it was two thousand years ago when it was incorporated in the great Epic.

It may be mentioned that the *Essays on the Gita* is his most read and popular work and has been translated into French, Chinese, Hindi, Marathi, Gujarati, Kannada, Tamil; more translations are being done.

Kapali Sastriar's *Gospel of the Gita* gives an outline of the argument and Pandit's *Light on the Gita* presents the thought of Sri Aurobindo topic-wise in a dictionary form. Anilbaran Roy's *Message of the Gita* in English (with the text) and his larger work with exhaustive commentary in Bengali are very popular.

SOCIOLOGY

Sri Aurobindo does not rest laying down a philosophy of divine realisation and in building a path to realise that Ideal. He knows that man does not live in isolation. Man is a unit of Life, a unit of Mind, organised in the universe. He influences and is influenced by the society in which he lives. How best to regulate this relation between the individual and the collectivity so that the spiritual evolution of man is best served? And what is really the nature of the collective evolution? In what direction is the collective society moving? Sri Aurobindo discusses these questions in the light of his perception of the spiritual evolution of the world and traces the gradual growth of human societies through several ages: the symbolic age, the typal age, the conventional age, the individual age, the rationalist age and the current subjective age opening to new horizons of the Spirit. He also discusses the manner in which the most fruitful balance can be struck between the needs of the individual for freedom and the claims of the society for its growth: he finds the level at which both the individual soul and the collective soul meet, the level of spiritual unity and observes that no solution, no panacea which fails to touch this source of truth can really succeed in solving this age-old problem which has worried so many social thinkers in the West. The series of essays he wrote on the subject in the *Arya* under the title *The Psychology of Social Development* have now been issued under a new title, *The Human Cycle*. This book is being translated into several languages.

Nolini Kanta Gupta's *Malady of the Century*, Kishore Gandhi's *Social Philosophy of Sri Aurobindo*, study modern developments in the context of this teaching.

THE IDEAL OF HUMAN UNITY

Sri Aurobindo also studies the development of human polity right from the beginnings of the formation of the tribe, clan, etc., up to the latest huge conglomerations of empires and commonwealths, and traces through all the historical processes one line of growth of humanity on the political level: an increasing association for common interests leading to the emergence of the State and the States in turn coming together in the form of federations and confederations, these again pointing to an eventual World Union. Inter alia, he analyses the various trends and movements, social, economic, political, idealistic and others with which the collective soul of humanity has been experimenting before deciding upon the final shape its body has to assume.

The World Union International, a non-profit and non-sectarian organisation, has been functioning for over a decade from Pondicherry with centres in different countries for the propagation and the establishment of this Ideal of the Union of the World peoples. Sri Aurobindo's work *The Ideal of Human Unity*, consisting of essays (seriatum) written originally during the years of the first World War and brought up to date by him in 1950 along with a post-script chapter in which he predicted in unambiguous terms the division of the world into two major blocks and the certain incursion of China through Tibet into India and into the South East Asia has been the object of study in many of the chancelleries of the world. It has been translated into French, Chinese, Hindi, Marathi, Telugu already.

INDIAN CULTURE

It was in December 1918 that Sri Aurobindo started a series of articles on Indian Culture under circumstances that are interesting. The well-known dramatic critic, Mr. William Archer, had just brought out a book condemning Indian culture lock, stock and barrel (under the title *India and her future*). Sir John Woodroffe wrote a spirited rejoinder entitling it *Is India Civilised?* This startling title set Sri Aurobindo on a course of exposition of the fundamentals of Indian culture. The series of *Is India Civilised?* were followed by another series *The Rationalist Critic on Indian Culture* which in turn were followed up by a massive *De-*

fence of Indian Culture. The whole series examined the broad motives of Indian culture, the developments in the civilisation based upon them and proceeded to expound in detail its essential character of life-embracing spirituality under different heads: Religion and Spirituality, Indian Art, Indian Literature, Indian Polity. The entire writings have now been issued under one connecting title *The Foundations of Indian Culture.* There is no peer to this book in its range and its depth and it is hoped that all who are interested in knowing the history and the future of Indian Culture will study this work.

Sisir Kumar Mitra has written a number of books in the light of this original exposition, notably *Resurgent India, Evolution of India, The Dawn Eternal* etc.

Sri Aurobindo's writings on Indian Nationalism are of course well-known. His writings in the *Bande Mataram, The Karmayogin, Indu Prakash* etc. are being collated and issued under suitable titles, e.g. *The Doctrine of Passive Resistance, Speeches, On Nationalism, Bankim-Tilak-Dayanand.* Particularly on the subject of Education, Sri Aurobindo has written with first-hand experience and these writings call for a revival of the basic values of the ancient system of education though in changed forms suited to the new conditions of the day. His *Brain of India, System of National Education, National Value of Art* are seminal books which if studied with attention could give much food for thought to those today who are concerned with the deterioration in the educational standards all over the world. We may mention in passing that the Mother's book *On Education* and the one on *Four Austerities and Four Liberations* are something unique in the field for the thoroughness with which she tackles the problem of education and invests education with an altogether new content and significance. According to the Mother, real education starts even in the pre-natal stage and continues up to the very day of death of the physical body. Experiments are being made on these lines in the International Centre of Education that has grown up in the Ashram where students and teachers from over fifteen countries in the world are participating in the project.

LITERATURE

Sri Aurobindo once observed that he was first a poet and then a patriot but never a philosopher. And, indeed, he was a poet from his very childhood. He started writing poems even as a student in England. But his literary career proper may be said to have started when he was in Baroda. For it was here that he wrote, or began to write, many of the narrative poems, plays and translations from the Classics. His plays have varied locales: *The Viziers of Bassora* with the aroma of Baghdad, *Rodogune* in the Syrian setting, *Eric* of Norway, *Perseus the Deliverer* of ancient Greece, *Vasavadutta* of mediaeval India are all classical dramas which have become very popular. There are a number of incomplete plays which we do not mention here. There is *Baji Prabhou,* a narrative poem, celebrating the Maratha bravery, *Love and Death* woven round the ancient love of Ruru and Priyamvada and a large number of a shorter poems and lyrics that have been issued in various editions. Most of his poems written in the Pondicherry period are spiritual in character: *Poems Past and Present, Ahana and other Poems, Last Poems, More Poems, Transformation and other Poems* etc. His translations include the *Hero and the Nymph* (rendering of Vikramorvasie in English verse), selections from *Ramayana* and *Mahabharata,* the *Century of Life* (translation of Nitishataka of Bhartrihari), *Songs of Chandidas* and *Poems from Bengali.* Some of his works, like the translation of Meghaduta have been unfortunately lost during his hectic political days. His essays on the art and style of *Kalidasa,* the genius of *Vyasa* and *Valmiki* are studies in depth and throw great light on the mind and soul of the Epic and the Classical Ages in Indian civilisation.

An original treatise of his on the theory of poetry, the course it has taken in English literature, the contribution of the Vedic seers to the evolving manifestation of the Poetic Word, the *mantra,* and the future of poetic expression, are the main topics in the *Future Poetry.* His greatest work in this line is of course the *Savitri,* which is the longest epic in English verse consisting of a little more than 23,000 lines. It is both a Legend and a Symbol. Adapting the story of Savitri-

Satyavan from the Mahabharata, Sri Aurobindo por-
trays the entire history of man in the cosmos, his
origin and his goal, the birth and the organisation of
the universe, the growth of Consciousness and its several planes or worlds through which the spiritual evolution of the earth-being proceeds, and much more.
Savitri may be described as a poetical rendering of the
Life Divine. Profound experiences of Yoga are described in a language and with a power that communicates the very experience to the awakened reader.
Savitri has been hailed as a new Veda of the New
Age.

Sethna's writings on *Savitri* and *Sri Aurobindo the
Poet*, Purani's *Approach to Savitri*, Prema Nandkumar's
doctoral thesis, *Study of Savitri* and Pandit's *Readings
in Savitri* (of which five Volumes are out so far) are
helpful for a proper understanding of the work.

Sri Aurobindo's Letters explaining his concepts and
technique in poetry have been issued in a separate volume, *Letters on Literature*. A distinct school of poets
has grown around him and their output is quite substantial. K. D. Sethna, Nirodbaran, Nishikanto, Nolini
Kanta Gupta are some of the well-known names in
this field.

BIOGRAPHY

Sri Aurobindo did not write any autobiography, but
a compilation has been made of Notes and Letters by

him bearing references to his own life and issued under the title *Sri Aurobindo on Himself*. And though he discouraged prospective biographers from writing upon his life, a number of biographies have been published in various languages. Mention may be made of *Sri Aurobindo: A Biography and A History*, by Dr. K. R. Srinivasa Iyengar, *Sri Aurobindo, the Hope of Man*, by Keshavmurti, *The Liberator*, by Sisir Kumar Mitra. Purani's chronicle of Sri Aurobindo's life events till 1926 is a useful source-book. Besides these, reports of *Talks with Sri Aurobindo* by Purani (three volumes) and by Nirodbaran (2 volumes so far) throw much light on Sri Aurobindo the man. Pandit's *Reminiscences and Anecdotes of Sri Aurobindo* is an interesting collection.

All this is about the literature by and about him so far published. Papers and notebooks are still being found on his shelves and they are under study. Letters are still being collected from various quarters and edited. Wide research is going on in different subjects following the trail blazed by the Master. A number of doctoral theses are being published from the various University centres in India and abroad on different aspects of Sri Aurobindo's thought, e.g. political, literary, philosophical, mystic.

Years and years ago poet Tagore said to Sri Aurobindo: "You have the Word and we are waiting to accept it from you. India will speak through your voice to the world, 'hearken to me'." The Voice has spoken; the New Age is being ushered in.

SRI AUROBINDO: AN ESTIMATE

The 15th of August, 1972, completes one century since the creative genius that is Sri Aurobindo came to this our earth — the chosen field of evolution in the universe. He came with a God-given mission. Even as a boy of eleven years of age, he had a strong presentiment that great changes were coming upon humanity and that he himself was destined to play a leading part in them. Some sixty years later, looking back on the events that had happened, the history that had been made, he observed how what had appeared to be impractical dreams, when he began life, had started realising themselves.

The first of them was the dream of a free India.

The part that he played in arousing the nation to the call of Mother-India in chains, his role in galvanising the political leadership and launching the country on the sure road to Independence, are well known. His services in awakening the mind of the nation to its priceless heritage — spiritual, cultural and social — and restating these fundamentals in clear terms for the regeneration of its life along the lines of its own temperament, are not less remarkable. He restored to the Indian a rightful pride in his heritage, chalked out the directions in which he must develop his life — individual and collective — in order to justify his title to the glory of that legacy and make of it a dynamic factor for the progress of the peoples of the world. He underlined the fact that the basic truths of Indian culture and civilisation are eternal, but they are to be recast in new forms from time to time in tune with the spirit of the Age. As long as the Indian people keep true to this demand of the Nation-Soul, their life is assured of continuity. That is how their civilisation and course of life have outlasted all others on this globe and shall do so in the future as well.

Spirituality has been the main fount of India's life-force, but it is a world-affirming spirituality, infusing with its dynamism all the branches of knowledge, all the fields of her expression. Sri Aurobindo has laid down the lines on which this mission of India is to be fulfilled.

Though Sri Aurobindo looked upon the freedom and development of India as crucial to the progression of the world towards its destiny, his vision embraced the other nations as well. Particularly he was concerned with the awakening of Asia, the mother of most civilisations, and the assertion of their freedom to progress by all the countries of this continent. He welcomed the rise of Japan, the gathering changes in China even as far back as the first decade of this century. He hoped that their resurgence would be in the moulds natural to their own genius and not in the alien forms of the West. At the end of the First World War he foresaw the definite emergence of Asia as a considerable force in the world situation and exerted himself in ways seen and unseen towards that end. Writing in 1947, he noted: "Asia has arisen; large parts are now quite free or are at this moment being liberated: its other still subject or partially subject parts are moving through whatever struggles towards freedom. Only a little has to be done and that will be done today or tomorrow." And true to the letter, Asia is politically liberated; economically it is being rejuvenated.

And more. Sri Aurobindo looked forward to a World-Union forming the outer basis of a nobler life for mankind. He welcomed all attempts, however half-hearted, towards this unification and himself wrote and worked at his own level for the unity of nations. He looked upon the League of Nations, the United Nations Organisation, as so many necessary steps forward and called for more radical steps for the realisation of Human Unity. He always stressed that the oneness has to be first promoted on the psychological level in which case alone the outer structure would become living and meaningful. He wrote two classics on the Psychology of social development and the growth of humanity towards the Ideal of Human Unity and these great works have influenced the higher mind of humanity in a definitive manner.

This awareness of oneness of the race, unity of creation, cannot really come from mental theorising or logical reasoning. It has to proceed from the deeper levels of the being, the spiritual. The world is rapidly developing in various dimensions, but its poverty in the one region that matters most, the spiritual, continues. Sri Aurobindo looked forward to the spread of spiritual knowledge from India to the rest of the world. For down the ages, India has been the home of spiritual experience at its deepest and also at its highest.

And in all ages her spiritual discoveries have reached and influenced men in countries beyond its shores. Sri Aurobindo resuscitated the comprehensive spiritual tradition of India from the debris and overgrowths that had covered its true visage, linked it with the findings of modern Science and established a positive spiritual Ideal of Perfection of Man. The movement of spiritual thought and life that commenced in the last century with the advent of Ramakrishna-Vivekananda gained immensely with the promulgation of the philosophy and practice of Life Divine by Sri Aurobindo and the world is currently receiving the rising tide of Indian spirituality. "Indian spirituality is entering Europe and America in an ever increasing measure. That movement will grow; amid the disasters of the time more and more eyes are turning towards her with hope and there is even an increasing resort not only to her teachings, but to her psychic and spiritual practice."

(Sri Aurobindo)

And the last crowning step is the acceleration of the next stage in the evolution of man. Sri Aurobindo and his radiant collaborator, the Mother, have devoted their entire lives on earth towards the accomplishment of this objective.

As is well known, Sri Aurobindo perceived that this world of ours is a developing progression of an unfolding Consciousness. Spiritual evolution is the process of this unfoldment. Consciousness, the *cit* as the ancients called it, is manifesting on this globe in developing forms, stage by stage. The stage of inert Matter was followed by the outbreak of Life; that in turn was succeeded by the formation of Mind; the next inevitable step, Sri Aurobindo points out, is the manifestation of the Spirit, the Soul, the Divine Mind which is a principle of Truth-Knowledge, Truth-Will, Unity. All evolutionary change and effort is inexorably moving in this direction. Man is on his way to becoming a God-man, a being with a God-consciousness of which harmony, peace, oneness are the natural workings. The global way of thinking that is now common in the higher rungs of humanity is a concrete evidence of this advancing change. Sri Aurobindo did 40 years of uninterrupted sadhana to hasten the advent of this rule of Divine Consciousness and the Mother has been currently engaged in establishing on earth the hold of this New Consciousness that promises nothing less than an unadulterated Life Divine to our distressed humanity. By his *tapasyā* to actualise this state of the Truth-Consciousness on earth, Sri Aurobindo has made it possible for man to achieve this Ideal of a divine kingdom in himself and in the race and built the path to this glorious fulfilment.

Well can he say:

To lead man's soul towards Truth and God we are born,
To draw the chequered scheme of mortal life
Into some semblance of the Immortal's plan,
To shape it closer to an image of God,
A little nearer to the Idea divine.

SAVITRI

SRI AUROBINDO
AND
HIS YOGA

PART II
Sadhana in Sri Aurobindo's Yoga

Introduction

THE immense range of the prolific pen of Sri Aurobindo is matched only by the Olympian quality of the writing that flows from it. He wrote his first poem in his eleventh year; his last writing, 'The Mind of Light', in his seventy-eighth. The subjects that received the alchemic touch of this divine man are varied: Art, Poetry, Criticism, Philosophy, Religion, Sociology, Polity, History, Yoga—all these are treated with a depth of insight and universality of outlook which bring to the fore their meeting ground in a commonness of purpose. Whatever the period, earlier or later, whatever the subject, the spirit that governs all his writings is the Ideal of Perfection of Man, the Gospel of Divine Life on earth. Whether it is the romantic dramas of the early years of his literary activity or the pungent editorials and fiery utterances during the political phase of his meteoric career or it is the metaphysics of his Teaching, the keynote of his writing is always the same—the divine potentiality of man.

And indeed, it could not be otherwise. For, the Truth he came to fulfil, the Ideal for which he devoted the major part of his life on earth is the possibility, nay, the inevitability, of a New Life for the human race. This consummation of the æonic labour of Nature in evolution is sought to be effected by a revolutionary precipitation of its process by which a new Consciousness shall manifest and impel the life on earth, bringing about a radical change in its character; in a word, deliver human life from the hold of Ignorance, Incapacity and Death into the freedom of a divine Knowledge, Power and Immortality.

Sri Aurobindo develops this theme and expounds it in all the ramifications of a metaphysical system in his basic work, 'The Life Divine'. The means for translating this Doctrine into practice and the experience which gives life to the theory, is described in his other great work, 'The Synthesis of Yoga'. How this urge in man for a total self-perfection is reflected in the development of society and how this ideal of self-fulfilment can be worked out in collectivity is shown in 'The Human Cycle'. 'The Ideal of Human Unity' traces the lines on which the far spread peoples of the globe are slowly but steadily moving towards an overt realisation of the Truth of Oneness that is governing their development from within, analyses the nature of the obstructions delaying the achievement and indicates the direction in which the solution is to be found.

Sri Aurobindo then proceeds to see how far this Knowledge of his perception and experience is

Introduction

consistent with the main spiritual and cultural
tradition of India and for this purpose takes up the
ancient texts of her Scriptures. He goes straight to
the core of the hymns of the Rig Veda, bares the
thought-structure that is embedded in them and
gathers in a methodical form the various hints
scattered all over these remnants of a rich hymnal
past, signposts of the inner discipline perfected by
the Rishis for their self-culture and development.
His findings are set forth in the series on the 'Secret
of the Veda' and in his translations of a large
number of hymns and commentaries on them, now
collected together under two titles, 'On the Veda'
and 'Hymns to the Mystic Fire'.

Similarly with the Upanishads. He translates
and gives a detailed exposition of the thought in
the Isha and Kena Upanishads[1] drawing attention
to the comprehensive character of their teaching
which embraces the whole world as a purposeful
manifestation of the all-pervading Brahman, Brahman that is Knowledge-Power-Bliss. He has besides
given free renderings of the Katha, Prashna, Taittiriya, Aitareya, Mundaka and Mandukya texts[2] and
annotated upon certain key concepts in the Taittiriya, the Chhandogya[3] and the Brihadaranyaka.[4]

Next, he takes the Gita which records a high
watermark reached by the turn for synthesis
characteristic of the Indian genius. He expounds
with a convincing thoroughness the manifold Way
prescribed in it for the application of the gains of

3

the Spirit to the dynamic side of life—activity—as also for the use of action for the growth of the being Godward. These brilliant 'Essays on the Gita' are among the most widely read of his writings.

In all these studies, be it noted, Sri Aurobindo does not rely on any of the extant commentaries for arriving at the import of the scriptures. His is a straightforward approach of an open mind and his conclusions are seen to be well tested on internal and circumstantial evidence of the texts themselves.

Besides these major sequences in his writings which we have dwelt upon elsewhere,[5] there is a large number of works,[6] smaller in bulk but not less significant for that reason. We propose to study some of these works, notably those which have an important bearing on the practical side, the Sadhana, of the Teaching of Sri Aurobindo.

And of them, naturally, first comes 'THE MOTHER'.

NOTES ON INTRODUCTION

[1] *Isha Upanishad, Kena Upanishad.*
[2] *Eight Upanishads.*
[3] Vide *Advent*, Vol. X, No. 3.
[4] *Sri Aurobindo Mandir Annual* No. 12.
[5] *The Teaching of Sri Aurobindo.*
[6] There is a considerable mass of poetry by Sri Aurobindo in English the most important of which is the Epic, *Savitri: A legend and a symbol*, in which he sketches the whole gamut of the spiritual adventure of humanity and embodies in it the course, the scope and achievement of his own mission for the transfiguration of mortal life into a Poem of Immortality. But this is a vast subject by itself and falls outside the limits we have set for ourselves here.

4

The Mother

THOUGH slender in volume, this work occupies
a key position in the Yoga literature of Sri
Aurobindo. For, it lays down in detail the steps of
the Sadhana, the indispensable discipline that is to
be practised if one is to realise the object of this
Yoga which is nothing less than the transformation
of human life into a divine living.

The task is formidable, indeed, impossible to
achieve by human effort alone. It is only the Divine
Shakti at work in the universe, in the Creation
projected by Herself and led by Herself for the
fulfilment of Her own Purpose, that can accomplish
it. She is to be invoked and in Her hands placed
the sadhana. But there are conditions in which
alone the Supreme Shakti will act.

There must be, in the first place, an *aspiration*
in you for the higher Truth. It is not enough that
the aspiration is there ; it must be intense, it must
pervade more and more all the parts of your being
so that the whole is afire with a live incessant call
for the Divine Power to manifest itself.

Consistent with this dynamic aspiration you
have to learn to *surrender* yourself to the Higher

5

Shakti. You must gather up all your movements and deliver yourself to the Power with a complete submission to its Will and command. The surrender must be active, cooperative, not tamasic and inert. There must be besides an exclusive self-opening to the Divine working and to no other. It defeats your purpose if you invoke the Divine Power and at the same time allow in you movements that are alien to the Truth of your seeking. At every step there has to be a *rejection* of all that proceeds from what is not the Truth, not the Light. The rejection has to be entire. There should be no acceptance or even sympathy anywhere in you with any element of falsehood and ignorance.

This triple labour of aspiration, rejection and surrender is the contribution demanded of you. For although it is true that it is the Divine Shakti who really carries out the sadhana in you, yet so long as you remain subject to the lower nature your personal effort is indispensable; you have to exert to overcome this nature. And in proportion as you rise above it and place yourself in the charge of the Higher Power, your effort is gradually replaced by the working of the Shakti. And there is no limit to the wonders that the Shakti, the Divine Grace, can effect in you. Only, from your side is asked a constant faith, sincerity and utter surrender. The more complete they are, the more secure the protection and sure the progress.

The ideal sadhaka is one who is conscious of

the Divine not only in himself but everywhere. All is Divine in origin and all has to be won back for the Divine, releasing it from the hold of the lords of Ignorance and Falsehood. Of the forces and powers put out from the Divine, the most usurped and the most misused are the forces of Wealth, Power and Sex. The seeker of the Integral Path has not to renounce but to exert and reconquer them, yoke them to the Purpose of the Divine. And this he can do only if he is free from the taint of desire and attachment, attains an equality of mind and purity of heart.

To be a true worker of the Divine, one needs to be totally free from desire and ego, the twin mainsprings of normal human activity. A perfect doer of Divine Works is one who is perfectly identified with the Divine Consciousness. But such an identification can only come as a culmination of a self-giving process. In the beginning of this sadhana, the sadhaka does the work that is given him as work for the Divine Mother. He seeks no personal gain. To do service to Her, to offer works to Her is its own reward. Her pleasure is his fulfilment. In time the sense of his being a worker gradually recedes and the consciousness of an instrument replaces it. His increasing devotion for the Mother brings about such an inner contact and intimacy that he has only to refer things to Her and he receives Her instant guidance. Not only guidance, but also the force to effectuate it. The

sadhaka begins to realise that all powers and
faculties are only channels for Her Force and
action. And as this closeness and identification
with the Mother increase in their pervasion and
intensity, the sadhaka feels no longer a worker or
a servant or an instrument. He feels and realises
in his being, that he is a child of Hers, truly a part
of Her Consciousness. All his movements are
consciously felt to be Her Movements. He is just a
mould of Her Knowledge, Her Force, Her Ananda.

Who is the Divine Mother to whom the seeker
is called upon to make a complete surrender and
who carries him safe in Her arms through the
perilous path? How is She felt and seen? How
does She work and pour Herself in the human
vessel? Sri Aurobindo reveals this Knowledge in
the last and the major part of the work which is
aptly described as the *Mātṛ Upaniṣad*. Here in one
matchless prose-poem winging out of his luminous
Seer-Vision, he lays bare the secret lore of the
Manifestation of the Divine Mother for the liberation and perfection of man and the revelation of
the Supreme on earth.

*　　*　　*

The Consciousness-Force of the One Supreme
Being is the Mother of all creation. For it is this
Divine Conscious Force, Shakti, that brings the

worlds into manifestation out of the Being, upbears and leads them in their career, in a word, mothers them. There are three ways of Her being in which it is possible to be aware of Her. She has three statuses.

Transcendent, She is above all the worlds, linking the Supreme Being to all creation. She it is who bears the Supreme in Her consciousness, calls and holds the truths to be manifested and casts them into form. All is Her Lila with the Lord.

Universal, She spreads Herself out as the substance and the soul of each universe of Her creation. It is Her presence that gives life and meaning to all, Her movement that gives the direction.

Individual, She embodies in Herself both the transcendent and the universal ways of Her existence and makes their Power operative here for the manifestation of the Divine in each individual form. She descends in person into the world of Ignorance in order to uplift and release it from the Falsehood and obscurity into which it has sunk.

The Divine Mother has many aspects, many personalities, that severally express the plenitude of Her oceanic Being. Of these, Sri Aurobindo points to the Four which have most to do with and are incessantly active for the evolution of this universe towards its destined goal of Perfection in the verities of Knowledge, Power and Ananda. They are Maheshwari, Mahakali, Mahalakshmi and Mahasaraswati.

Maheshwari is the Personality who presides over the infinite expanses of Knowledge. She builds the human soul and nature into the Divine Truth and opens out our summits into the splendours of the supreme Light.

Mahakali embodies an all-effectuating Power and Will. Hers is the divine Warrior-Force that smashes all obstruction and speeds upward human aspiration and effort.

Mahalakshmi is the soul of all Beauty and Harmony in creation. It is She who manifests the hidden Bliss in life and prepares the receptacles for the divine Ananda.

Mahasaraswati holds in Herself an inexhaustible capacity for flawless work and exact perfection. Nearest of the Four to physical Nature, She is most concerned with organisation, execution and construction, all of which She carries out with a thoroughness that is integral.

Sri Aurobindo's narration of the characteristics of these Four Powers of the Divine Mother, their ways of working, their conditions to manifest, their mission of love and labour for man, forms one of the most enthralling pieces of the spiritual literature of all time.

There are other Powers too of the Divine Mother. But they are more in the background and will manifest only when these Four have established and founded their harmony. Then will their supramental action be possible which alone can finally deliver the thrice bound nature into the dynamic freedom of the Spirit.

If you seek this transformation, be surrendered absolutely in the hands of the Divine Mother; be always conscious in every part of your being,—mind, soul, life, the very cells of the body-consciousness—of the presence of the Mother and the workings of Her Powers; and be plastic to Her touch, ever pliant to comply with the demands of Her Force, to be shaped at all moments and in all movements in the mould of Her choice. For only so can the supreme Truth, Light and Ananda be brought down into this world of falsehood, obscurity and suffering, and human nature transmuted into a divine supernature.

The Yoga and its Objects

THERE are yogas and yogas. Each yoga has its own means; some base themselves on the physical organism, some on the life-dynamism, some on the emotional, others on the mental faculties, and yet others seek to combine in their method one means with another. But all of them, broadly speaking, have one aim viz. to heighten the state of one's being above and beyond the normal bounds of the body and life and attain a release into a freedom of self-existence or non-existence—*mukti*. The yoga of which Sri Aurobindo speaks here, however, is of a different kind. It is distinctive in its aim and distinctive also in its means. The object of this Yoga is not liberation, *mukti*, but fulfilment, *sampatti*. Fulfilment of what? of the Will of God in Creation. And what is that Will?

The Divine has projected the universe out of His own Being with a purpose. That purpose is to manifest Himself, His inalienable nature of Existence, Consciousness and Bliss, *saccidānanda*. It is the aim of our Yoga to work out this Supreme Will by the liberation of human life from the holds of Ignorance, Limitation and Death and its transformation into the divine nature of Knowledge, Infinity and Immortality. The whole of man,—not the mind alone, or the soul alone,—is to be taken up and subjected to the transforming change. All the faculties of the being are to be yoked to this One Purpose. This is the means, and this the goal of our Yoga which is indeed a Purna Yoga, the Integral Path, as it includes all of man and consequently all of life in its comprehensive scope. To be sure, such a grand objective as this is beyond human means to reach. It is only the World-Power which has initiated the Movement that can lead it to its victorious culmination.

In the context of this aim of our Yoga, liberation of the individual soul, personal *mukti*, ceases to be the sole object. It is indeed indispensable, but only as a necessary and inevitable step. For without the central transcendence of the triple rule of the lower nature governed by Ignorance, no divine change is possible.

*   *   *

The first truth the sadhaka of this Yoga has to perceive is that all is the Divine, the One Brahman. He permeates all orders of existence. He is there in every creature, in every point of Space and in every moment of Time, supporting all as the *sad ātman*, an impersonal Self. All are Names and Forms on the bosom of this Self.

This realisation of an impersonal divine Existence deepens further into a second realisation in which one sees the Divine not only supporting and containing but also embodying itself in all things. Not only are all things in the Self, but the Self too is in all of them. It is That which makes the Names and Forms alive and real.

And there is a third, the crowning realisation to follow : above all there is the fact of an infinite Divine Personality, the Supreme Purusha, who transcends both the world of Names and Forms and the Impersonal Atman supporting them. It is He who has put out this universe from the infinitude of His being and who presides over it in the Lila of His manifestation.

The whole world-existence changes its hue. It is no more a battlefield of contraries ; it is realised to be a variegated self-extension of the Divine Being in His waves of Light, Beauty and Bliss which strike under certain conditions as their very opposites. From Him radiate all these multiplications in Creation and it is in Him also that we find our oneness with others. He is the Lord in whose sovereign sway the sadhaka has to awaken and grow. It is to this Supreme Person that you have to deliver yourself for the completion of your life's mission.

If you would have the Master assume the reins of your being in his celestial hands you must surrender yourself to Him absolutely. Absolutely : neither in the mind, nor in the heart nor even in

14

the body shall there be any reservation. All is to
be given in a sacred offering. True, complete surrender is not possible in a day. Still one can begin
with a whole-hearted *saṁkalpa*, an attitude, a will
to surrender imposed on the entire being. No
egoistic demand, however faint, no personal preference, however masked, shall be allowed to taint
the purity of this consecration. All dualities must
be renounced and all existence embraced as an
expression of the One Divine. If you thus give yourself up wholly into His hands, the way is clear for
the working of His Lila through you and in you.

When this is done there is no need of a formal
discipline, *kriyā*. For it is the Divine who takes up
and effectuates the Yoga. And besides, the utmost
that man could do by his own effort is nothing
compared to what is possible for His mighty
Shakti.

Once the initial surrender to the Lord is made,
the next step is to stand aside and observe the working of His Shakti. The complex movements of its
process, now taking up a few ends here, now
changing over to other threads there, unsettling the
established round of nature,—all these and many
more appear to land one in the very heart of chaos
and bewilder the anticipating human mind. A
quiet strong faith in the intelligence and the ultimate effectivity of the Higher Power at work is
required of the sadhaka. Whatever is done within
or without, it is the work of the Shakti offered to

15

the Lord as a *yajña* of which the sadhaka is only the *yajamāna*. As the *yajamāna*, he holds the *ādhāra*, sees the sacrifice progress and tastes the fruit given to him. Not involved in the movement as a doer, he perceives the true nature and the extent of his *ādhāra*. He awakens too to the yet concealed regions of his being where the divine part of himself dwells—regions where abound masses of knowledge and the seas of *ānanda*—and he learns to let their revelation glide into an overt participation in his life-progression.

*　　*　　*

The sadhana of Purna Yoga has many lines of movement. But the most effective start is made by offering to the Divine the fruit of your actions. To give up the fruit of action means you do not perform actions for the particular fruits you expect of them; you do what comes to you ordained by the Master, *kartavyam karma*, regardless of the results. Whatever the results, they are given by God and you receive them with trust in His Wisdom.

Next, you surrender not only the fruit but the actions themselves to the Lord. You realise that you are not the doer. You perceive that it is really Prakriti, the executive Power of the Divine that is doing all action at the command of the Lord. It is He who determines the action through your *sva-bhāva* and it is the Prakriti who executes it. Once you realise this truth in the depths of your being,

neither action nor the results of action can bind
you. Sri Aurobindo speaks of three stages in the
growth of this knowledge :

first, when you surrender the initiative to the
Master of your being and act as He directs ;

second, when you believe that in the heart of
all beings there is God moving them by his Maya
of three Gunas and are able to perceive that you
are really not the worker at all but it is the machinery of the three Gunas that does all works. By
steady dissociation from the Gunas you stand above
them in your central poise, the Purusha, and in
time the Prakriti too will be free from their mechanical hold ;

third, when the very Gunas, of which the
Prakriti is constituted, undergo a transforming
change. Sattva passes into Jyoti, pure illumination,
Tamas into Shanti, infinite Calm and Rajas into
Tapas, a divine Force. Whatever action proceeds
from such a foundation of a new harmony will be,
indeed, an undeflected expression of the will of the
Purusha, one with the Will of God. A vast and
mighty Force will be found moving and acting in
you, possessing your mind, your heart, your very
body, and you yourself will be one centre of the
divine Dynamism.

It is indispensable for this liberation that you
should be totally free from desire, *spṛhā*, which
creates longing and attachment to things, from
duality, *dvandva*, which forges on the being the

17

clamps of attraction and repulsion, love and hate, from egoism, *ahaṅkāra*, which creates a false identification with things resulting in one's bondage to them. All these take their characteristic expression in the workings of the three Gunas of Tamas, Rajas and Sattva,—the most dangerous being the deceptive formulations of the Sattva Guna,—and are the enemies of self-surrender.

These processes are worked out by the Divine Shakti in its own rhythm with its own pace and stress varying with each individual need. All that is demanded of you is a continual remembrance, a constant assent to the workings of the Yoga Shakti with an unshakable faith and a vigilant perseverance. For the path is long, the Goal is high. It is nothing less than the acceleration of centuries of evolution into a few years of Yoga, the transformation of your entire human nature into a divine nature. Yet it is not your own puny will and effort but the infinite Shakti of the Almighty that is charged with the task and whatever the time taken, whatever the failings in the instrumental nature, its fulfilment is inevitable. The reliance here is on God and God does not fail even though man in his stumbling steps may.

These, then, are the four aids for the *siddhi* of this yoga :

S'āstra, the teaching of *sarvam khalu idam brahma*, All is Brahman, and *ātma samarpaṇa*, total self-surrender to the Lord of all ;

18

The Yoga and its Objects

Utsāha, zeal in pursuing the path with constant assent and remembrance;

Guru, the Teacher who is God Himself or the person who embodies Him to the disciple;

Kāla, Time, the duration of which is ultimately decided in the all-knowing Wisdom of the Master of all Yoga.

The Superman

FOR a sadhaka of the supramental Yoga, as
    indeed of all Yoga, it is indispensable to have
beforehand a right understanding of the nature of
the Goal of the path he is to tread. He should
know, as precisely as possible, the full content of
the Ideal, its implications immediate and eventual,
so that no effort is misdirected or wasted, no turn
taken that would defeat the very purpose of the
Journey.

The aim of this Yoga is to exceed the boundaries of the imperfect mind in man and to enliven
in him a principle which is free from the limitations
of mind, a faculty which is above the mind,—the
supermind. Man is to grow into a superman.

Now what exactly is meant by superman?

It goes without saying that a superman is not,
as is commonly conceived or misconceived, simply
a glorified edition of the ordinary man. A man
whose powers and capacities are raised to an
uncommon degree, towering high above his less
fortunate fellow beings, dominating them by virtue
of his superior might—this is the figure of the superman popularised by vitalist thinkers like Nietzsche.

Such a man, it will be noted, remains still a man. Only his faculties have an enlarged sway; they continue to be centred round his ego which is now much more exaggerated. He is a veritable titan, an Asura, whose role in the cosmic evolution is happily past. The superman of our conception is one who has cultivated and perfected in their fullest amplitude and height the essential powers of his being in all its ranges of body, life, mind and soul but at the same time has purged himself of all deformations of ego and ignorance and passed into godhead. He has risen above the reign of nature and enthroned himself in the freedom of the soul from where he governs her activities. He is the master of his own being, *svarāt*.

He too governs the lives of others but in another sense. He is one with them in the secrecies of their being, feels their heart-beats as his own and pours his energies for their advancement. Freed from the bonds of the separative ego, he expands in his consciousness gathering into its fold the wide universe around. He holds all in his clasp, not of power, but of love. He receives in his illumined being the movements of those around and returns them uplifted and charged with his transmuting vibrations which exert an incessant pressure on his environs moulding them in the likeness of the Truth of his living. He is the world-ruler, *samrāṭ*.

He is no more subject to the law of Division which is characteristic of the rule of mind. In him the several principles of Existence e.g., Knowledge, Love, Power, Unity, do not clash and seek to suppress each other in their drive for exclusive expression as they do in the mind-governed domain of man. They develop, each into its fullness, and find their completion in the fulfilment of all. All see each other as the common petals of a budding rose. The many notes struck by them fall into a rich harmony and he reproduces in himself the rhythms of the cosmic harp in the hands of God.

This and no other is the significance of the superman. To this end must man work with a singleness of purpose, exercising his will enlightened by the growing light of the soul at every step, to eliminate all that belongs to the lower order of life and to choose what leads to the higher, however difficult and arduous the course may be. But is he free to choose? Is man not, more truly, a leaf driven hither and thither by the gusts of universal forces? Is he not just a creature under the goad of Karma, Fate, forged by himself and by others?

* * *

There is, says Sri Aurobindo, a truth in Fate, in determinism. There is also, he adds, a truth in Free-will. Both are two movements of one Cosmic Energy put out by the Divine Shakti at work. The universe is an expression of a Will and all in it follows the lines of that Will for the execution of its Purpose. In this sense all is determined. But the Will works through a hundred currents of its own formulation as Power, Energy that is many-tiered. In the individual it works most effectively through his sense of freedom, freedom to choose and act. This freedom of the individual is a device of the All-Will to effectuate itself. The will of the individual is a segment of the Universal Will and what it works out is ultimately just what is assigned to it in the larger Plan of the One Will.

And yet, within certain limits the individual is free to choose. Even the compulsive factors in Nature, Heredity and Environment, which Modern Science emphasises to underline the rigid law of causation governing this material world, are only elements that are provided by an All-seeing Intelligence for the free choice of the soul at every graded step of its evolutionary career. Once chosen these factors come into their own operation, call it by whatever name you will. But it is the soul that chooses initially; it is again the soul that chooses its own destiny in the future by means of the Karma it puts out at every moment consciously.

The individual will is a part of the Universal Will and the secret of progress lies in the discovery of harmony between the two. As long as one chooses to act by one's own ego-will regardless of the demands of the greater Will there is friction, struggle and even catastrophe. But as one learns

to identify oneself and make oneself Its instrument
the friction dissolves and a harmonious working is
ensured. To awaken to this role of the instrument
is then the first necessity.

*   *   *

To the seeker of the truth of this Manifestation
of the Divine, all work is work for the Divine and
by the Divine. He perceives that for each work
there is the Master of the Work, the Worker and the
Instrument. He knows himself to be neither the
Master nor the Worker. He is only the instrument.
He equips himself as a ready and willing instrument
whose sole aim is to serve as a perfect channel for
the divine execution and whose whole joy lies in the
privilege of being so chosen. He learns to feel the
inmost law of his nature, sets all the members of his
being in tune with this demand of the soul and
grows into a joyous conscious instrument of the real
Worker who is none other than Nature.

That Nature is All-Nature of which his own
nature is a special movement. Hers is the one
Force that works and effectuates simultaneously in
the individual and in the universe. The sadhaka
awakens to this fact of One Nature within and
without and gradually identifies himself with the
infinite Force of All-Nature. As his consciousness
widens and deepens in this Knowledge, he becomes

24

aware that it is not for herself that all work is done by Nature but for the One who is her Lord.

He discovers the poise of the Lord on the heights of his being even as he comes to recognise the dynamics of the Executrix-Nature in his own.

It is only when he knows and begins to live this triple truth of the Instrument, the Worker and the Master in his own being that man shall have the full joy of work, his share in the Lila of Manifestation.

The Letters

OF all the writings of Sri Aurobindo the most
important from the standpoint of *sādhanā*,
practice of yoga, are his Letters. His correspondence
covers a large variety of subjects : Yoga, Philosophy,
Literature, Art, Occultism, Astrology, Sociology,
International affairs etc., etc. Aspirants for spiritual
life, practitioners of his Yoga within the Ashram
and outside, put their difficulties and doubts before
him and sought his guidance and help. Experiences,
visions, dreams were submitted for interpretation.
Learned men and professional philosophers posed
searching queries on fine points in the metaphysics
of his gospel of the Life Divine. Disciples who
found poetic inspiration welling up in them in the
course of the Yoga sent their efforts for his
scrutiny. At times even mundane matters and
opinions of men in public life were placed before
him for comment. And so it went on. He used to
deal with most of the letters himself, meticulously,
and for a considerable number of years it took a
good many hours daily[1] to deal with all this volume

[1] *Vide* Sri Aurobindo's own remarks in this connection :
" The volume of correspondence is becoming enormous and it takes

26

of correspondence. At its peak there were more than a hundred letters every day. Many of his letters in reply were later compiled, either in full or in extracts, under suitable titles and issued in book-form from time to time.[1] Recently a comprehensive collection of his letters dealing with Yoga has been brought out in the Sri Aurobindo International Centre of Education Series.[2] And it is with the letters on Yoga that we are concerned in our present study.

Most of these letters were written to sadhaks of the Integral Yoga, in response to their queries and seekings for guidance. Developments and difficulties in the day-to-day course of the sadhana were placed before the Guru by the disciples and he wrote to them explaining, clarifying things, and

---

me all the night and a good part of the day—apart from the work done separately by the Mother who has also to work the greater part of the night in addition to her day's work."

" I have to spend twelve hours over the ordinary correspondence, numerous reports etc. I work three hours in the afternoon and the whole night up to six in the morning over this." (*Sri Aurobindo on Himself and on the Mother*).

[1] *The Riddle of this World, Lights on Yoga, Bases of Yoga, More Lights on Yoga, Elements of Yoga, Letters (First, Second, Third and Fourth Series), Life-Literature-Yoga, Correspondence with Sri Aurobindo* (by Nirodbaran), I & II series.

[2] *On Yoga*, Vol. II, Tomes 1 & 2.
This is, naturally, not yet exhaustive ; letters are still being collected and edited. They are being published, as they get ready, in some of the periodicals of the Ashram, viz., *The Advent, Mother India*, Annual Numbers of *Sri Aurobindo Circle*, Bombay.

what is more, he used such occasions to communicate his special help, through the medium of the written word and otherwise, in order to meet the situation and speed up the progress. And these communications were a source of inspiration and helpful pointers on the Path to others as well. As he himself says :

"If I have given importance to the correspondence, it is because it was an effective instrument towards my central purpose—there are a large number of sadhaks whom it has helped to awaken from lethargy and begin to tread the way of spiritual experience, others whom it has carried from a small round of experience to a flood of realisations, some who have been absolutely hopeless for years who have undergone a conversion and entered from darkness into an opening of light . . . for the majority of those who wrote there has been real progress. No doubt also it was not the correspondence in itself but the Force that was increasing in its pressure on the physical nature which was able to do all this, but a canalisation was needed, and this served the purpose.[1]

It is not necessary to add that the letters were not answers in the usual intellectual way but 'answers from higher spiritual experience, from a deeper source of knowledge and not lucubrations of the logical intellect trying to co-ordinate its

[1] *Sri Aurobindo on Himself and on the Mother.*

ignorance'.[1] In them we see Sri Aurobindo not in
the role of the Prophet of the high Philosophy of the
Life Divine, nor even as the High Priest ushering in
a New Age by means of a Poorna Yoga holding in
itself all the essentials of the past spiritual effort
of humanity and forging a new Dynamism, but as
the Master with a supreme understanding of human
nature and its countless foibles, with an endless
compassion for its cry for help, ever ready to
support, guide, and lead the seeker with an infinite
patience along the steep path of Yoga. Nothing is
too small, nothing too profane to claim his attention. His Yoga touches life at every point and no
part of it is outside his scope. As a result, we
have in these Letters a most comprehensive body of
practical knowledge not only invaluable for those
living an inner life of the spirit but an equally reli-
able guide for a better, harmonious and enlightened
conduct of the general life.

*   *   *

Though it is true that each individual has his
own line of spiritual growth and what is valid for
one need not be so for another, yet there are certain
fundamental truths which are common to all types
of sadhana. And this is particularly true in the

[1] *Sri Aurobindo on Himself and on the Mother.*

case of sadhaks of the same Yoga. Whatever the individual variations in the experience of the Yoga-process, the broad governing Truth is the same. It is with this background that we have to approach the Letters of Sri Aurobindo for a helpful study of his Yoga.

The Object
of Integral Yoga

TO begin with, what is the object of the Integral Yoga developed by Sri Aurobindo?

The object is, first, to grow from the normal limited human consciousness into a higher, wider Divine Consciousness.

Next, this Divine Consciousness with all that it contains,—Peace, Light, Joy, Knowledge,—is to be progressively brought into a direct functioning in our external nature in order to totally change that nature into its own higher illumined term, the Supernature.

The purpose of this transformation is to manifest the Divine in our life. And of this manifestation our personal liberation is a part—only a part, though an indispensable one. This manifestation of the Divine in our life implies a realisation and a sequent radiation of the Divine Consciousness not in the soul alone but equally in all the different parts of the being. What is aimed at is a complete union with the Divine on all the planes of one's being. The mind, the life, the body, the soul, all must be equally filled with the Divine Presence and

SADHANA

be effective centres for the outpouring of the Divine Power in the universe.

Or, to put it differently, the Integral Yoga has three clear objects in view :

First, the realisation of the Divine within one-self—the individual realisation.

Next, a felt seeing of the One Divine all around in the universe, the Divine which is identical with one's own Self—the cosmic realisation.

And third, an ascension into an order of the Reality which stands above both the individual and the universal manifestation, but bases them both —the transcendental realisation.

Each of these realisations must be attained and integrated within one's being so as to be simultaneously active and the miracle of the triple manifestation of God[1] is repeated in every individual frame : each man grows into his godhead.

It may be asked what the special feature and necessity of this Yoga is. After all God is One and there are a thousand paths to reach Him. What does it matter which path you take ? What is important is that you reach Him whatever be the path.

DISTINCTION FROM OTHER PATHS

Generally speaking, the goal of all the paths of Yoga is *mukti*, liberation. The world is a transient phenomenon, or an illusion ; if it is not totally

[1] Individual, Universal and Transcendent.

32

an illusion, it is definitely an inferior order of existence.[1] Limitation, incapacity and death are its badge. The one aim of the awakened man must be to get out of this round of pain and pleasure, life and death and effect a release into a blissful or an ineffable Beyond, call it Brahman, call it Nirvana. But in Sri Aurobindo's Teaching the Universe is as real as the Divine of which it is a willed Emanation. It is not a falsity imposed upon the Truth of Brahman. Nor is it something inferior. It is a self-formulation, *as yet imperfect*, of the manifesting Godhead. And the sole object of the Yoga of Sri Aurobindo is to complete this outflowering of the Divine Consciousness on earth. It aims at a fulfilment of the Divine Intention, first in the life of the individual and then in the life of the collectivity. It gives a meaning to the life on earth which is not a whit less significant—perhaps it is more—than life in the heavens in the scheme of Creation.

Aiming as they do to reject life in this apparently transitory and unhappy world, the other yogas generally seek to realise the Self, the Atman, behind or above the mind-led life of the body, and through it disappear into the Vast Impersonality of the Great Self or into Nirvana, extinction. That is to say, the way is one of withdrawal from the line

[1] Or, in conceptions like the Christian, life on earth is only a preparatory stage to an eternal existence elsewhere—heaven or hell—after death.

33

of manifestation of which this earth forms a crucial part. The Integral Yoga on the other hand, keeps to the evolutionary line of ascent in the Manifestation. The self within is to be realised; but that is only the first step. After attaining to union with this self, one has to effect an enlargement of the consciousness to arrive at an identity with the larger Self, the Universal Atman and embrace the totality of Existence supported by It. This is further followed by an ascension into the dynamics of the Divine Knowledge, Power, Bliss—an aspect which reveals itself to the seeker beyond the summits of the spiritualised mind, on the planes of the Supermind. And it is these verities of the Divine Existence that justify the human aspiration for perfection of life on earth. It is they that shall bring into overt expression the full Nature of the Divine, hitherto at the back of the manifestation, and confirm and complete the movement for the revelation of the Divine Truth in human life.

The aim is different; the direction is different; the process too is different in important details. For instance, in the other yogas one is not called upon to subject one's nature to a transmuting change. It is enough if the nature is silenced or modified enough to prevent its being a drag or a block to the inner progress of the soul godward. Even after the realisation is achieved, no special attention is paid to the outer nature. It goes on in its mechanical round carried on the impetus of past

Karma and drops away at the death of the body leaving the soul completely free. But it is not so in this yoga. Each part of the nature, submissive or recalcitrant, has to change; it has to leave its moorings in ignorance and allow itself to be recast into its higher potential. The whole of the external nature, including the physical body, must be made supple and pure enough to hold and respond spontaneously to the Divine Consciousness housed in it.

Again, in this yoga, there is no suppression or stoppage of the flow of life energies or the legitimate activity of the senses. They continue to function in full but in an enlightened spirit imbued with the growing Light, Power and Delight of the Divine Truth. Not asceticism but a radiant plenitude of life is the Way. In the ways of the Vedanta, it is enough for the inner Purusha to attain union with the Divine; in those of the Tantra, what is required is an effective identification with the Shakti, individual and cosmic, and that gives the release. But here both are combined. The Realisation in the consciousness of the Purusha has to spread to the Prakriti. The Purusha regains his mastery over Prakriti and both together lift their human embodiment to an altogether new altitude in the scale of human Evolution.

Basic Requisites
of Integral Yoga

TO take up this yoga, one must first feel the need
for it. There should be a *Call* for the higher
life. And the call must be genuine, must proceed
from the depths of the being. Impulsions from the
surfaces of the mental or of the vital personality,
either as a result of some dissatisfaction in life
or ambition—under whatever camouflage—could
never be a sufficient reason. They do not last for
long and there comes the inevitable flag, after the
initial push is spent out. One must feel a real
need to change the ordinary way of living into a
higher. There should be a thirst for the Divine as
the fish, in the apt imagery, thirsts for water. The
demand must be of the soul with a sustained pressure on the mind and the vital to seek and share
the change. Again the novice must make sure of
the type of spiritual life for which he has affinity.
For this Integral Yoga there must be an aspiration
in the whole of one's being, not only in the mind
and the soul, but in the life-being and the body
too, to be reborn in the dynamic truth of the Spirit
and to participate in the Divine's manifestation. If

the call is only for Mukti, liberation, then there is
no need to choose this difficult path of transformation. There are other traditional paths for that
purpose.

Next is *Sincerity*. And by sincerity is meant a
constant readiness and effort to lift up all the parts
and all the movements of one's being, in consonance
with the truth of one's seeking. It is not enough if
the sincerity is there at the centre, in the mind or in
the heart. It should spread to all the parts of one's
being so that each acts spontaneously on the same
basis and for the same aim. The whole being must
be true to the Ideal it has set out to realise. Nothing
foreign to that should be allowed to touch, much
less express itself in any of its thinkings or doings.

There must be *Faith*, faith in the reality of
the Divine, faith in the Path that leads to the Divine,
and faith in the Grace that carries one to the Goal.
Here too it is not enough if there is only a belief
or a certain adherence in the thought i.e. the mind.
There is required an entire faith, a dynamic convic-
tion in all the parts of one's being. Sri Aurobindo
speaks of four kinds of faith : the mental faith which
dispels all doubts and prepares for true knowledge ;
the vital faith which automatically repels onslaughts
of the adverse forces and builds up an effective
instrumentation of the divine Will and action ; the
physical faith which sustains the body amidst all
its tribulations of suffering, illness and inertia and
silently prepares for the reception of the higher

consciousness in the material base; and lastly the psychic faith which draws a direct touch of the Divine Influence and leads to a joyous surrender to and intimacy with the Divine.

And of course there must be an *Aspiration*. The aspiration for the Divine has to be active, growing, setting aflame each centre of the being so that in due course the whole system is one tongue of Agni reaching out to the Heavens Supreme. This aspiration, to be effective, must needs be accompanied by a corresponding will to translate it into action. This conjoint movement manifests itself in the mind as a thirst for and growth into Knowledge, in the vital being as an urge shaping into a dynamic activity dedicated to the Divine, in the heart as a welling up of the emotions of love and devotion, all in adoration of the Divine. Even the body calls for and yields to a settling calm and peace in its very texture so as to form a firm pedestal for the rising structure.

All this is rendered possible by another means, *Surrender*. Surrender is a willed delivering of oneself to another, here the Divine. In this Yoga, starting from a part which most easily tends to so surrender itself, the movement gradually spreads over to the other parts making them all fall in line, so that the whole of oneself is placed in the hands of the Divine in absolute trust and confidence. This surrender is of two kinds, passive and active. It is active when the individual will is sought to be harmonised and identified with the divine Will at every step—this is what is called consecration—and there is a conscious effort to accept only what is divine and reject what is undivine. It is passive when no will is exercised, but the entire being is kept in a state of readiness to be acted upon by the Divine Will. This latter way is more difficult and unless one· is very vigilant one gets bogged in tamasic inertia or becomes a plaything of the forces of the lower nature.

That brings us to the next requisite, *Vigilance,* vigilance to spot out the opposite and wrong currents as they try to enter, to feel the right and upward movements as they set in and to tend them in the proper direction. This is indispensable so long as the sadhana has not been completely taken charge of by the Higher Power and personal effort has its part to play. Once the direction is taken up by the higher Agency, there is an automatic action of the psychic being within replacing the labour of mental vigilance.

For success in any spiritual life, especially in a Yoga as this where one aims to participate in the dynamic manifestation of the Divine, it is essential that the *ego* must be dissolved. Ego is a false front of the real individuality within and unless that is removed the true self cannot come into its own. Human ego has many disguises, many centres of operation and aggrandisement. There is the tamasic ego of wallowing in inertia, weakness and ignorance in a spirit of loud helplessness, a vital or rajasic ego of the sense of one's power and dominion, a sattvic ego of one's superior wisdom and moral righteousness, even a spiritual ego of sainthood. Each and every one of these forms of ego must be exposed and broken. This is a preliminary and yet a fundamental step to be taken before one can be secure on the path. A full recognition of one's limitations, awareness of one's imperfections, and a becoming humility before the Vastness of the Divine that seeks to manifest, are of great help in the elimination of the ego which is truly a formidable enemy of the soul.

These are the main requisites for sadhana on the part of the individual. His personal effort must base itself and proceed on these lines, for personal effort there has to be in the beginning and for a long time, till the initiative passes from him into the hands of the Guiding Power; even then, a continued state of receptivity and constant assent to its workings by the sadhaka is demanded. All these, however, constitute only one side of the endeavour. For, whatever may be the position in disciplines like the Advaitic or the Buddhist, in this Yoga the main burden rests with the Divine Power to whom an entire surrender is made. It is the Shakti that has first to assent to the sacrifice, the Divine Grace that has to accept and second the effort of the aspirant. That Grace is to be invoked and waited upon. For ultimately it is not the personal exertions of the human will but the uplifting move and the transforming touch of the Divine Grace that carries one over every obstacle and steadily changes the lower nature into the higher. And the Divine Grace is here manifest in the benign Person of the Guru, our Lord Sri Aurobindo and the Blissful Divine Mother who are pouring out in their compassion streams of Grace in abundance like the sempiternal Indra of the Veda raining the plenteous Waters of Heaven.

There have been disputes among scholars whether it is *tapasyā*, personal effort, that achieves or it is really the Grace that effects the result. In Sri Aurobindo's Yoga there is no room for any such doubt. Both are necessary; they are two sides of the working Truth. Divine Grace, surely, but for the Grace to be fully manifest the recipient should be ready. His being has got to be prepared, made pure, supple and sufficiently strong to receive, contain and collaborate with its workings. Otherwise the Breath of Grace will just pass by awaiting its Hour in the future. As the Mother says : "For transformation, Grace and aspiration are equally important. Grace comes first but if aspiration does not answer to It no progress is possible."

Foundations of Sadhana

ONE can begin the sadhana in any part of the being that is more awake than the others and seeks a higher direction. In some it is the heart that is astir and longs for the Divine Beloved; for them the most natural way is the Way of Love and Devotion. In some it is the mind that is ardent and searches for a Truth that is more satisfying than any it has known thitherto; for them is the Way of Meditation and Knowledge. In others it is the will, the life-dynamism that is dissatisfied with the normal round of activity and seeks to yoke itself to a higher Purpose and serve the Lord of All; for them is the Way of Works.

But whichever the Way one takes to in order to transcend the ordinary nature of humanity and grow into the heights and expanses of supernature, it is essential that the foundations of the sadhana are laid firm. Unless one prepares the base of the *ādhāra* strong enough to bear the incessant pressure of the Yoga Force at work for change, for growth, for reconstitution of the very texture of the being as in our Yoga, there is every danger of failure or breakdown on the way. The ordinary mind and

the vital nature of man are apt to lose their balance
and go off at a tangent once they are released—in
the course of yoga—from the limitations to which
they are normally subject; they may get overwhelmed by the descents of joy, power and light
that greet the yogin on the path. The physical body
itself, unless it is freed of its obscurity and rendered
supple, may not respond pliantly to the demands
of the Yoga-Shakti. To avert these dangers it is
indispensable that the sadhaka first lays a strong
foundation for the structure to come.

The very first step in laying the proper foundation, says Sri Aurobindo, is to acquire a Quiet in
the being. Quiet means a state of mind in which
there is no restlessness, no movement of anxiety or
similar emotion which keeps a constant tenseness
in the being and to that extent interferes with the
opening of the being to the Higher Consciousness
and obstructs the smooth and conscious reception
of the incoming vibrations of the Higher Force or
the outflowings of the soul within.

This quietude of the mind, *acañcalatā*, is to
be acquired, built up with vigilance and will. It can
be said to be established when there is no habitual
restlessness, no incessant movement keeping the
mind in a whirl. Though a negative condition, it is
the first step leading to the next, the Calm, *sthiratā*.
Calm is a more positive state in which there is a
kind of tranquillity which is not disturbed by
movement on the surface. Disturbances may come

and pass but they move on the surface; the mind is serene. Sri Aurobindo describes two kinds of Calm: the negative calm where there is no contrary movement; the positive calm which solidly resists all movements that seek to disturb.

A still more positive condition is when there is entry of Peace, *śānti*, in the being. It carries with it a sense of solidity, harmony and deliverance with a quiet Ananda permeating its vibrations. In such a state there can be no real disturbance which can affect the secure poise of the being.

The being is to be gradually taught to grow into these conditions of Quiet, Calm and Peace. Unless it frees itself from its habitual turmoil and naturalises these into its system, there can be no secure holding of the riches of the Spirit which one calls down into oneself by aspiration and will and which the Grace sanctions.

The most effective way to begin is mentally to conceive a Silence which is at the back of all movement. After all, thoughts are not the texture of the mind. Thoughts pass, other thoughts come and they too flit across some silent and immobile background of the mind. A repeated suspension of the thought-movement, and an increasing awareness of the Silence behind, effects the needed opening and the Silence begins to take hold of the mind. It is in this condition that Calm and Peace settle themselves. Here too, there are two kinds of silence. One, in which there is absolutely no movement in the inner consciousness; there is no reaction at all to activity in the external being; this is the passive silence. The other is the active silence in which from out of the Silence there goes out a powerful force of action without leaving a ripple within.

For true Peace to settle in the being there must be this stillness, the silence which prepares a state of utmost receptivity; it keeps the vessel empty. But this peace is not static. It is active and spreads to the other parts of the being as they begin to accept it, though initially it may enter through the mind. It has a purifying action wherever it goes and thus builds up a developing condition of purity which is an indispensable factor for progress in sadhana.

Purity is an equally essential part of the foundation. Naturally, by purity is not meant physical cleanliness. Nor is it only a moral rectitude of the kind spoken of in the Dharma Sastras. Purity, in Sri Aurobindo's sense, means an exclusive opening to the Divine alone; it implies the total rejection of all influences alien to the Divine. A sole fidelity to the Divine is what purity means in our sadhana. And Peace helps in the growth of this purity inasmuch as disturbing and foreign movements are automatically rejected from a state of Peace. Peace admits only those movements which are akin to its nature, nourish it and thrive in it. Further, inner Peace lessens the necessity of outer contacts and minimises the intrusion of external influences.

Next comes Equality, *samatā*. The normal
human mind and vital nature are always apt to
identify themselves with men and events, forces and
circumstances, as they impinge upon the person,
and get lost in the rush of their emotions and
passions. For a sadhaka it is necessary that he
should detach himself from the current of happen-
ings; he has to learn gradually to stand back from
the rush of Prakriti and observe things aloof from
them. That way he acquires a dispassion, a growing equanimity which faces men and events in
the world without getting helplessly involved in
them. All contacts are received in an equable and
unmoved status by the being and the utmost is made
of each circumstance for an ordered and rapid
growth of the evolving consciousness.

It is of course difficult to attain to this state of
calm equality within a short time. A fund of
patience and a steady will, persistent in the face of
all opposition and difficulty, to acquire and make
this inner equanimity a natural poise of the being
is demanded of the sadhaka.

And lastly there must be a spiritual atmosphere
in which the sadhana can thrive. If one can get it,
for instance, in the environs of the Guru, nothing
could be better. If not, one must create the spiritual
air around oneself and live in it. And that is
possible because the atmosphere one carries is
always a reflection of the state of one's inner
consciousness.

46

The Way of Works

ONE cannot but work, declares the Lord in the Gita. At every moment of our life we work in some way or other; we put out some energy consciously or unconsciously in the field of Karma. And where there is work there is usually a motive, a propelling factor that operates ceaselessly till the object is achieved and another replaces it. Normally the motive for work is based upon one's ego, self-interest, self-preservation, self-aggrandisement, and even when it extends beyond the range of one's personal self, it is still for interests related to the larger extensions of that self in the family, the society, the nation etc., or it is for the expression and affirmation of one's own ideas and ideals. Work so motivated and dictated by the demands of the ego continually forges fresh chains of Karma that keep the soul perpetually bound. For this reason, most spiritual disciplines counsel a gradual dissociation of the Purusha from the round of works, leaving the irreducible minimum to be performed by the mechanical Nature, Prakriti. In our Yoga, however, works are recognised as a God-given means of evolution and self-expression and valued as such. It is the motive that is sought to be changed. The usual impulsion based on the ego of the individual is to be replaced by a motive that derives from a deeper or higher origin, the psychic or the spiritual being. In this Path, works are directed to the Divine, performed for the Divine and even originated by the Divine. The individual remains but an instrument, a channel. Work is first used as a means for the establishment and the growth of self-dedication and consecration to the Divine and then utilised as a field for the expression of the Divine Consciousness that is being gradually realised and imbibed by the sadhaka in the course of his sadhana in works.

In order to convert work into a means of sadhana one begins by offering to the Divine the work that falls to one's share. Once it is dedicated to the Divine, work acquires a sacred character. It cannot be done in a light manner ; sincerity demands an appropriate order of application. An offering to the Divine has to be necessarily as perfect as possible and commensurate with his devotion ; there is an earnest attempt on the part of the sadhaka to do the work in a spirit of loving consecration. Every little part of it gains importance, no detail can now be left out imperfectly done. Further, it is no more the kind of work that truly matters but the spirit in which it is done. As the spirit of consecration grows, there is a happiness in the being, a stream of delight from the emotional and the psychic being converting the whole working into a rite of joyous progression in the Pathway to the Divine.

And in this process of doing one's best to make of work a worthy offering to the Adored, there is an automatic concentration of faculties and convergence of energies towards the One to whom the entire work is consecrated. Of course all this is not done in a day. It is not at once easy to remember continually the Divine to whom the offering is made. One forgets again and again and the mechanical habit of working asserts itself. Sri Aurobindo states encouragingly that to start with, it is enough to remember before the work is begun and to remember again with gratitude after the work is done. In between there are moments when one remembers; these should be steadily increased; if necessary, one can inwardly withdraw for a moment now and then, remember and renew the offering. If the initial will for consecration is sincere, one finds in the course of time that there are, as it were, two parts of oneself: one part engaged in work and the other silent, remembering the Divine. This calm and quiet being comes forward at moments when there is a suspension of the external preoccupation; but it should be possible for the sadhaka to be more and more aware of its supporting presence even during activity. Gradually, increasingly, one comes to experience that the whole of oneself is

SADHANA

this quiet and gathered being with only its frontal part doing the work.

This is the beginning. The work is offered to the Divine, but not the results ; they are sought after still on the basis of desire. The next step is to offer the fruits too to the Divine. Let the results be what the Divine determines, let me work irrespective of what they might be, leaving it to Him to make of them what He will. That is the attitude to be adopted by the sadhaka. If sincerely accepted and cultivated, this attitude gradually eliminates the claim and the domination of ego and desire and promotes a certain equality in the mind. For once both the work and its fruits are offered to the Divine, there is no straining for a particular personal result, no agitation of anxiety or fear of reverse ; whatever the results they are taken as indicating the Divine Will. The human will becomes only the servant of the Divine Will.

To be the servant of the Divine is only the first step. To be an instrument is the next. For this purpose the sadhaka has to invoke the Divine Shakti to take up the work and do it through him. And for this to be possible there are a few minimum conditions to be fulfilled. In the first place, there must be a sufficient degree of purity in the being, especially in the vital and the mental energies ; the claims and preferences of the ignorant mind and the habits of the ego-ridden life-being should not be allowed to interfere with the guidance and the

50

working of the Higher Force. There has to be a steady and effective elimination of these impurities from the system. A sufficient measure of Equality and Quiet in the mind, in the face of all likes and dislikes, all contradictions and oppositions that assail the worker, is indispensable and that can be developed only on the basis of a strong Faith, faith that all is determined by the Sole Divine and in spite of appearances all leads in sum to the result intended by the Divine. Only in such a state of quiet faith can one become aware of the presence and working of a Higher Shakti, the Divine Consciousness and Force. And becoming aware, one has to open oneself—in the static as well as in the active condition—to that Consciousness and to no other influence. Then the Force to which one opens oneself begins to act, first in moments when one is receptive, then in stretches of receptive periods and then longer and longer. There is not only a constant guidance and impulsion to do what is to be done, but also a vigilant and forceful pulling back from what should not be done. The human will and energy are taken up by the Shakti which makes them its channel and through them executes its purpose. All the while, it will be noted, the human consciousness goes on receiving the impacts and the pressure of the Divine Consciousness and Force; on the human side from below there is a rigorous discipline processing the system in the way of concentration, purification, dedication and receptivity to the Divine. All work becomes a sadhana to grow into the rising altitudes of the Divine Consciousness and receive the incoming Force and Illumination in one's own person.

Work is not only a means of ascent to the highest but more. Work is simultaneously a means to express what one acquires by way of enlightenment of will and power, increasing purity of motive and illumination of energy. In short, work becomes a field to bring out the inner gains and confirm them in the outer nature also by accustoming its faculties to express them infallibly. Further, once the individual is equipped as an instrument, the Divine Force that acts need not be limited in its dynamics by the imperfections of its nature. It can act in its own full power using the instrument as a readied medium. It may also—and usually does—train and perfect the instrument by acclimatizing it to the workings of its higher nature and naturalising in it the vibrations and movements of a higher Knowledge and Power. The sadhaka develops into a potent centre for the greater radiation of spiritual energy in the world.

The Way of Meditation

IT is possible to train the being to tune itself to the workings of the Divine Consciousness by another means, *dhyāna*.

Dhyana, commonly translated as Meditation, is of several kinds only one of which can be truly called Meditation. Sri Aurobindo analyses these different forms of Dhyana into four main kinds. There is first, meditation (*manana*) which is a dwelling of the mind on a line of thought or series of ideas constituting a single subject. The mind is allowed to flow into a channel of thought-activity centred around the object of meditation, which may be a Knowledge-Idea — say, the Divine as omnipresent, the Divine as one's own highest Self, the Divine as an Impersonal Power, the Divine as a Personal Deity with several attributes — or simply a Call to the Divine. The second is contemplation, a more concentrated direction of the mental faculties on a *single* Idea or Image or object. As a result of this concentration there arises in the mind, naturally, a knowledge of the object contemplated upon. There is a third kind, the Dhyana of self-observation, in which one stands back from the

53

running activity of thoughts and only observes the nature of one's mind as shown by the thoughts. The fourth is the process by which the thoughts are steadily rejected and the mind kept more and more free from the turbidity of thoughts so as to provide a more or less empty vessel in which the Higher Consciousness may settle itself ; this is the Dhyana of liberation, liberation of the mind from its mechanical and inferior movements into purer altitudes giving it the freedom to think or not to think, the power to choose its thoughts or go beyond them.

Each of these forms of Dhyana has its own value in spiritual life. The individual chooses that which is most natural to him. It is also found in the course of sadhana that the same line of Dhyana may not be suitable at all times. Different Dhyana-processes may be called for at different stages of development and one should be supple enough to use whichever method is the most helpful during the period.

The central principle of Dhyana, it will be observed, is to summon the various faculties of the being, particularly the mental forces, which are usually spread out in innumerable directions, and gather them round the object of one's quest. Indeed, in an ideal condition the entire being stands naturally so gathered and mobilised around the Truth of its seeking all the time. But a long prior discipline is necessary to train the being in this direction and to accustom it to function in that poise for longer and longer periods before it settles in that position normally. And this discipline is what is called Dhyana, Meditation.

There are certain conditions which are very helpful in the beginning, external and internal. There should be, in the first place, a reasonable measure of solitude, a seclusion where one could be by oneself and meditate without fear of physical intrusion or interruption by others. The next condition is that the body must be trained to take up a position that is most helpful for the purpose of meditation. That position is ideal in which the body settles into a state of gathered immobility freeing the rest of the being from the pull of the physical frame and providing for it a firm and stable base. The sitting position is the best for in that one can continue the course of meditation for longer stretches of time undistracted by restlessness or tiredness in the body. The sitting position in which the spine is kept erect and the chest, the neck and the head held up straight is the best posture as it promotes stability and a healthy coursing of vitality in the body infusing fresh currents of life-energy in the mental and *prāṇic* organisms which are the leading participants in the meditation.

The very first difficulty one meets with the moment one begins to meditate is the rush of thoughts. Thoughts crowd in such a bewildering profusion that it looks as if there are more thoughts during meditation than at other times. But this is

SADHANA

not quite so. The fact is, normally, men are so preoccupied with many other things that they are not conscious of the innumerable thoughts floating on the surface of the mind. When one prepares for meditation the mind is focussed in a narrower circle and the flow of thoughts comes to the notice more prominently than ever. Now there are ways of countering this invasion of thoughts.

One can stand back from the waves of thought and observe them without sanctioning or participating in them. There is no effort to reject or fight them. One simply stands back as a witness. Gradually for want of support from the active mind the thoughts begin to dwindle and peter away. Another way is to treat the thoughts as coming from outside and vigilantly check them when they try to enter the mind. Each thought is to be so detected and thrown out before it comes in or as soon as it is discovered. A third way is to treat the thoughts as foreign, as coming from Prakriti and for oneself to stand in the poise of the witness Purusha, without sanction, without approval or disapproval, aloof. This leads in time to a kind of bifurcation, a division in the mind — one part is quiet and watches, the other is the scene of crossing thoughts. It is possible afterwards to impose the quietude of the witness part on the part involved in the thought-movement. Yet another way is to ignore the movements of thoughts on the surface of the mind and to go within with a will, pursuing the

56

object of meditation. This succeeds to the measure
of the interest aroused in the mind : where it has
interest there the mind turns. The best method,
however, is to remember and invoke the Silence and
Peace that stands at the back of all thought and
movement. Whether at the back of our mind or
behind the universal movements there is a supporting Silence, a Calm, a Peace. And the sadhaka
should learn to mentally envisage it, invoke it
and gently lay himself open to its entry. In
course of time, this Calm and Silence makes
itself felt and once it enters the mind, in whatever
layer, the end of the rule of thoughts begins. It
is this Silence and Peace that is to be regarded,
concentrated upon, ignoring the activity of the
surface mind. Sri Aurobindo points out that it is
easier and more natural to let this Silence take hold
of us than for us to enter into it. And as the Silence,
the Peace, settles in the being, the consciousness gets
readied to receive and assimilate what comes from
above or within and opens to the reign of the Divine.
The turbid contents of the human vessel—passions,
desires and their reactions—are steadily replaced
by a quiet joy, enlightened emotions and increasing
purity.

The success of the meditation depends largely
upon the sincerity and strength of the aspiration
behind it. It is not duration but the intensity of
the aspiring consciousness that is important. The
Mother once observed that three minutes of intense

SADHANA

aspiration is worth much more than hours of stag-
nant meditation. Fatigue is to be avoided at all
costs : for with it concentration loses its power and
the mind jades. Sri Aurobindo advises relaxation into
meditation instead of concentration in such cases.

That brings us to other difficulties usually
encountered in meditation. Frequently one is overcome by sleep. However, this sleep, it must be
remembered, is not the usual kind of sleep. As a
result of the pressure to go within, the consciousness as it withdraws from the external world
tends to lapse by habit into sleep. But it is
only a part of it that so sinks into sleep; if there
be sufficient fire of aspiration, the larger part of the
consciousness is seen to be luminously active within,
below or behind the layer of sleep. If the sleep were
of the ordinary tamasic variety, it would not be
possible for the body to hold itself for long in the
erect posture of meditation.

Then there are the obstructions of forgetfulness, inertia and absorption into the mechanically
repetitive habits of the mind ; they are best negatived
by constant vigilance, ardour and a strong will in the
effort. There are also the obstacles of restlessness,
impatience, over-eagerness and violence of effort
which soon tire and bring in depression. These are
to be eliminated and replaced by patience, persist-
ence and a quiet aspiration.

During meditation the consciousness (not
merely the outer mind which is only a segment of it)

58

is withdrawn from its usual activity of ceaseless reception of and response to external contacts and turned to its own larger expanse, whether inwards or upwards, which is more open to and in a way in contact with the Divine Consciousness. So turned and tuned, the limited human consciousness is exposed to the touches and workings of the Force of the Higher Consciousness which prepare and precipitate its change from the lower into the higher, from the human into the divine nature. This concentration of consciousness is usually done either in the head or in the heart. When the natural inclination is to seek the Divine within oneself, the concentration is done in the heart centre (in the middle of the chest, the cardiac centre) with a strong aspiration for an opening inward and realisation of the Divinity seated deep within. When the urge is to rise in one's consciousness above the bounds of the mind or to invoke the descent of the Peace above the mind, the concentration is done in the head. Such a concentration is indeed strenuous but the strain begins to disappear as one learns to 'lift the concentration above the brain-mind'.

Thus meditation puts the being of the sadhaka in a condition of increasing and conscious receptivity to the workings of the Yoga Shakti. As it deepens there is even a total forgetfulness of the external environment and outer nature. There is a steady settling in of peace, joy, light, knowledge and other inalienable powers of the Higher Consciousness in the inner mind and being of the practicant. In most lines of Yoga this condition, experienced uninterruptedly in the hours of Samadhi —the crown of Dhyana—, is stabilised and organised into a state of liberation in the inner being to the exclusion of the rest of oneself—the external nature in its triple formulation on the mental, vital and physical levels—under the rule of Ignorance. But in the Integral Yoga of Sri Aurobindo, care is taken to relate the inner realisation at every step to the outer nature. The ordinary consciousness which is sought to be completely stilled and immobilised into the state of Samadhi in the older Yogas, the Patanjala Yoga, for instance, is here quieted and into that quietude are brought down the powers of the Higher or Deeper Consciousness to change its very nature. The condition of receptivity and illumination realised during meditation is consciously prolonged even during other hours and made the base of all movements of active life. As one progresses inly, further effort is made to communicate and dynamise in terms of life the golden gains of Meditation.

The Way of Love

LOVE is the easiest key to open the Gates to the Divine. This is a love that wells up spontaneously from the depths of the heart, oozes out from every pore of the body at the very thought of the Divine Beloved. It is a love which is very different from what we call by the same name in human relationships. What passes for love in the ordinary world is really no love at all but a mixture of desire and self-interest masquerading under as attachment, affection, love. Its root is ego and the moment the return it expects fails to come there is a revolt; love is on its way to turn into hate. The love that we speak of in Yoga is totally different. And there too, usually, it is not there in the beginning but comes as a culmination of the movement of devotion, Bhakti.

Even Bhakti, says the Scripture, is not always an unmixed offering of the emotions to the Divine. There is a Bhakti of appeal for succour from distress, *ārta*; there is a Bhakti propelled by desire seeking its fulfilment from the Divine, *arthārthī*; there is a Bhakti which is the outcome of the thirst for knowledge of the Divine who attracts but is still

61

Unknown, the Bhakti of the *jijñāsu*. There is also a Bhakti which is the result of the Knowledge, *jñānam*, that the Divine is the Sole Lord of All. Whatever the nature of the initial Bhakti, it should be taken as a starting point and an effort made to gradually cleanse its content, purge it of its grosser motives and turn it more and more into purer channels leading towards selfless love. In this the seeker is helped by the very nature of Bhakti which whatever its original motive, apparent or real, comes into its own as it grows in his being and raises him repeatedly to the high peaks of utter gratitude, pure love and clean aspiration, all of which are doors of entry into the realm of Love.

The first movement of Bhakti is one of *adoration*. Usually this takes the form of some kind of external worship of the adored. The devotee tends to express his feeling of submission and reverence through physical means which is natural to a mind that normally dwells in the world of the physical senses. This worship has indeed its preparatory value. But to be truly effective in opening a way of contact and communication with the Divine who is worshipped, this outer mode of attendance must correspond to an inner feeling, a glad movement of surrender, a dependence felt within. The outer should be a means of expression, a support for the growth of an *inner adoration*. The inner gives life to the outer.

With the birth of this inner adoration Yoga

may be said to begin in right earnest. An inner life begins to take shape. The sense of submission and waiting upon the Divine with devotion—implied in the act of adoration—has certain practical consequences. There is an automatic action to keep the temple of one's being clean for the Divine. Thoughts and feelings turn into movements of seeking and prayer. The external life too comes to be moulded in tune with this inner ordering.

There grows an effortless *consecration* to the Divine who is sought after. And a necessary part of this consecration is self-purification. It is an inner purification: a relentless elimination of all that is contrary to the spirit of one's central endeavour, an abstention from contacts, physical, mental or vital, which tend to draw away from or contaminate in their results the purity of the seeking, a soulful tenderness and receptive expectancy which draws the Divine to reveal itself to the seeker.

All the faculties of the mind, its thought, will, imagination, are turned towards the Divine. The mind is gradually orientated towards the Divine on the wings of the heart's love. Once smitten with Love for the Supreme Beloved, the mind loses interest in the objects that held its attention before and turns to centre itself wholly round the Divine. Till that stage is reached, one may initially take the help of an Image or a Name to gather the energies of the mind and focus them on the Object of the seeking. Once the mind is trained to so concentrate itself, the image or the name gradually melts into the Reality, the Divine Personality they stand for and the consciousness of the seeker is engulfed in the Revelation. There is also the well-known process of hearing the glories of the Divine, *śravaṇam*, constant thinking of them and of Him whom they celebrate, *mananam*, and the settling of the mind on the Divine who is so adored, *dhyānam*. When this last condition deepens, the consciousness passes into an ecstatic trance, *samādhi*, in which the individual completely loses himself in the Object of his adoration.

Sri Aurobindo draws attention to the distinction between this Samadhi of the God-lover and the Samadhi of the discriminating Jnanin. The Bhakta's is an ecstatic experience, not the still and silent contemplation of the Jnanin of the Way of Knowledge. Here one does not pass into the Being of the Supreme but calls the Divine into oneself. Not peace of unity but bliss of union is the crown in the Way of Love.

Not only consecration of the mind but consecration of the body also. All outpourings of the will and energy are offered to the Divine. Here too there is a difference between the methods of dedication of the path of Bhakti and of the path of Works. In the latter it is the individual will that is taught to tune itself to the Higher Will of the Divine. The fulcrum is the will. But in the way of Devotion the motive-spring is love. Love is the dominant force which turns all action flowing towards the Divine as its dynamic outreaching. Work becomes at once a means for the expansion of love and a channel for the expression of love for the Divine in His manifold Becoming.

Thus does Bhakti, starting from whatever motive, gradually gather strength, shed its earthly dross and acquire the character of heavenly love which ever glows in the deepest centre of man, his psychic being. Sri Aurobindo enjoins upon the seeker to try and awaken this psychic element in himself so as to bring into operation its natural power of love which when it comes into its own, can alone by itself burn away the impediments and heal the imperfections in his nature. And Love has this supreme power, for in its pristine nature, it is the most divine dynamis in creation. It is, we may say, the yearning of the Divine in the individual form towards its Source, the Parent Divine Above. When the veils that cover it are removed and it is allowed to come to the front, there is no withstanding its imperious surge. From a spark it grows into a flame setting the whole being on fire for union with the Divine.

For the seeker of the Integral Yoga it is indeed not enough to realise this truth of love and union in his psychic depths alone. The union in love is to be realised in his other parts as well. They too have a secret aspiration and intention to participate in the bliss of union and contribute their characte-

65

ristic powers in manifestation to add to the varied delight of the Union. The vital has a dynamic role to play; especially the higher vital with its large capacities for self-giving, heroism and mighty effectuations. The physical body too has its elements of stability and beauty to serve as a moving Temple of Love Divine.

Conclusion

THESE are broadly the three lines on which this Yoga can be pursued. Each one takes a particular faculty or power of the being for its base and fulcrum, and as the Yoga develops, that basic power is cultured and gradually raised to its highest potential. But in actual practice it is found that these different processes are not exclusive. Each one as it proceeds, touches and sets into motion the other processes also. Thus the doer of dedicated Works, serving the Lord with his will yoked to the supreme Will, finds a spontaneous welling up of devotion and love for Him on whom all his activities are centred. So also is the Bhakta moved to express his inner surrender and adoration of the Lord in the entire submission of his will to the Lord's and all his outer actions become movements of consecration. So again does the sadhaka of the way of Meditation and Knowledge find that his increasing awareness of the presence of the Divine everywhere fills him with an irresistible sense of wonder, devotion and surrender in which his dynamic will becomes a joyous slave of the Divine so perceived. It is not that these developments are successive to each other. They are more or less simultaneous.

SADHANA

The sadhaka of the Integral Yoga chooses that part of his being which is most developed and ready and starts with the mode of Yoga natural to it. Thus if he is preponderantly of a dynamic and expansive nature, he finds it natural to begin with his will disciplining itself in the way of Works; if he be primarily an emotional type and the heart is his central station of living he finds his way already selected for him; he takes the way of Love; or if he be more quietistic in temperament and accustomed to follow the lead of his mind, the *buddhi*, then the way of Meditation and Knowledge is the obvious line of progress for him. But human nature is not made of the mind alone or the heart alone or the will only; the being is complex and what moves one part or one power of it has its repercussions on the others in varying degrees. And especially in a Yoga like the Integral Yoga where the being in its entirety is exposed to the uplifting and transforming action of the Higher Shakti, it is most natural that alongside the main current of advance and progress, though in a lower key, other parts begin to respond in a contributory way and slowly gather strength to function on their own.

Whatever the starting-point and the main direction, the sadhana proceeds through four distinct phases. There is, first, a marked separation from the surface movements of the external nature and a growing awareness of a deeper and larger consciousness that makes itself felt. Thoughts, impulses, volitions begin to arise and function from this inner level of the being and the more one remains awake to this emerging expanse within the more is the normal human consciousness replaced by a deeper yogic consciousness. This new consciousness has to be brought into fuller sway, naturalised and made effective at all times.

As this is done with vigilance and patience, one tends to go still inward and discovers the real centre of life within, the soul or the psychic being, which is truly a portion of the Divine within oneself. The next phase in the sadhana is to draw this psychic element forward, evoke it in all the movements of mind, will and body, refer to it constantly, and thus organise one's whole life around the psychic. This operation is called the psychicisation of the being i.e., imparting the character of the psychic to all the rest of oneself, placing the whole of the being under the governance of the Psychic Monitor.

This gradual shift of the centre of one's consciousness from without to deep within has its repercussions in the opening of the higher levels of the being freed from the confines of the individual formulation. There is a natural extension of one's consciousness and a beginning of a living sense of unity with all in the universe around. One awakens to the throb in the universal Life of the same Divine Shakti that pulsates within oneself. This widening of the being goes on under the impulsion of the psychic *puruṣa* till the whole of the universe is embraced.

That is not all. There is an effortless move upward too. The consciousness in the mind either ascends to the regions above it or opens itself to the descent of what is above. These are the altitudes of the spiritual mind, the higher mind, the illumined mind, the intuitive mind etc., each of which has its own characteristic consciousness deriving from the Truth in manifestation, which is assimilated by the aspiring mind. There are several realisations of a transforming nature that the mind undergoes in its ascension. Thus for instance, above the boundaries of the Intellect, one is greeted by summits where all is silent : a Silence that impinges upon the consciousness as alone true and against the background of which all else appears temporary, fleeting and illusive. This is the belt of experience which has given rise to most of the theories of the illusoriness of the world and the sole reality of a Nihil, Nothing, an Ineffable. But that is not the final terminus.

Beyond the Silence are the glories of the *parārdha*, the Higher Worlds of Knowledge, Power and Joy with their corresponding principles and powers formulated in the individual. These are the planes of spiritual felicities which stir into life in the sadhaka. The vistas that open are endless, from plateau to plateau, say the seers of the Veda. Farthest known are the worlds of Sat, Chit and Ananda. They too can be realised, not merely in some Transcendent beyond the universe, but here in the individual they can be embodied and manifested. And ultimately that is the aim of this Creation. The immediate aim of the Yoga of Sri Aurobindo, however, is to rise above the bounds of the human mind, scale the heights of the higher, the illumined, the intuitive and still higher grades of the Mind and arrive at the Gnosis, the plane of Knowledge-Will which is the plenary manifestation of the Divine in its creative poise. That is the objective. The way to reach and receive it in one's own being and consciousness is the Yoga we have sketched out whose central process is best recapitulated in the words of Sri Aurobindo:

"A disclosure from within or a descent from above are the two sovereign ways of the Yoga-Siddhi. An effort of the external surface mind or emotions, a tapasya of some kind may seem to build up something of these things, but the results are usually uncertain and fragmentary, compared to the result of the two radical ways. That is why in this Yoga we insist always on an 'opening'—an opening inwards of the inner mind, vital, physical to the innermost part of us, the psychic, and an opening upwards to what is above the mind—as indispensable ·for the fruits of the sadhana.

"The underlying reason for this is that this little mind, vital and body which we call ourselves is only a surface movement and not our 'self' at all. . . . The real Self is not anywhere on the surface but deep within and above. Within is the soul supporting an inner mind, inner vital, inner physical in which there is a capacity for universal wideness and with it for the things now asked for—direct contact with the truth of self and things, taste of a universal bliss, liberation from the imprisoned small-ness and sufferings of the gross physical body. . . . It is according to our psychology, connected with the small outer personality by certain centres of consciousness of which we become aware by Yoga. Only a little of the inner being escapes through these centres into the outer life, but that little is the best part of ourselves and responsible for our art, poetry, philosophy, ideals, religious aspirations, efforts at knowledge and perfection. But the inner centres are for the most part closed or asleep—to open them and make them awake and active is one aim of Yoga. As they open, the powers and possibilities of the inner being also are aroused in us, we awake first to a larger consciousness and then to a cosmic consciousness; we are no longer little separate personalities with limited lives but centres of a universal action and in direct contact with cosmic forces. Moreover, instead of being unwillingly play-things of the latter, as is the surface person, we can become to a certain extent conscious and masters of the play of nature—how far this goes depending on the development of the inner being and its opening upward to the higher spiritual levels. At the same time the opening of the heart centre

releases the psychic being which proceeds to make
us aware of the Divine within us and of the higher
Truth above us.

"For the highest spiritual Self is not even
behind our personality and bodily existence but is
above it and altogether exceeds it. The highest of
the inner centres is in the head, just as the deepest
is the heart ; but the centre which opens directly to
the Self is above the head, altogether outside the
physical body, in what is called the subtle body,
sūkṣma ś'arīra. This Self has two aspects and
the results of realising it correspond to these two
aspects. One is static, a condition of wide peace,
freedom, silence : the silent Self is unaffected by
any action or experience ; it impartially supports
them but does not seem to originate them at all,
rather to stand back detached or unconcerned,
udāsīna. The other aspect is dynamic and that is
experienced as a cosmic Self or Spirit which not
only supports but originates and contains the whole
cosmic action—not only that part of it which
concerns our physical selves but also all that is
beyond it—this world and all other worlds, the
supraphysical as well as the physical ranges of the
universe. Moreover, we feel the Self as one in all ;
but also we feel it as above all, transcendent,
surpassing all individual birth or cosmic existence.
To get into the universal Self—one in all—is to be
liberated from ego ; ego either becomes a small
instrumental circumstance in the consciousness or

73

even disappears from our consciousness altogether. This is the extinction or Nirvana of the ego. To get into the transcendent Self above all, makes us capable of transcending altogether even cosmic consciousness and action—it can be the way to that complete liberation from the world-existence which is called also extinction, *laya, mokṣa,* Nirvana.

"It must be noted however that the opening upward does not necessarily lead to peace, silence and Nirvana only. The sadhak becomes aware not only of a great, eventually an infinite peace, silence, wideness above us, above the head as it were and extending into all physical and supraphysical space, but also he can become aware of other things—a vast Force in which is all Power, a vast Light in which is all Knowledge, a vast Ananda in which is all bliss and rapture. At first they appear as something essential, indeterminate, absolute, simple, *kevala* : a Nirvana into any of these things seems possible. But we can come to see too that this Force contains all forces, this Light all lights, this Ananda all joy and bliss possible. And all this can descend into us. Any of them and all of them can come down, not peace alone ; only the safest is to bring down first an absolute calm and peace, for that makes the descent of the rest more secure ; otherwise it may be difficult for the external nature to contain or bear so much Force, Light, Knowledge or Ananda. All these things together make what we call the higher spiritual or Divine Consciousness. The psychic opening through the heart puts us primarily into connection with the individual Divine, the Divine in his inner relation with us; it is especially the source of love and bhakti. This upward opening puts us into direct relation with the whole Divine and can create in us the divine consciousness and a new birth or births of the spirit.

"When the Peace is established, this higher or Divine Force from above can descend and work in us. It descends usually first into the head and liberates the inner mind centres, then into the heart centre and liberates fully the psychic and emotional being, then into the navel and other vital centres and liberates the inner vital, then into the Mula-dhara and below and liberates the inner physical being. It works at the same time for perfection as well as liberation; it takes up the whole nature part by part and deals with it, rejecting what has to be rejected, sublimating what has to be sublimated, creating what has to be created. It integrates, harmonises, establishes a new rhythm in the nature. It can bring down too a higher nature until, if that be aim of the sadhana, it becomes possible to bring down the supramental forces and existence. All this is prepared, assisted, farthered by the work of the psychic being in the heart centre; the more it is open, in front, active, the quicker, safer, easier the working of the Force can be. The more love and bhakti and surrender grow in the heart, the more rapid and perfect becomes the evolution of the sadhana. For the descent and transformation imply at the same time an increasing contact and union with the Divine.

"This is the fundamental rationale of the sadhana. It will be evident that the two most important things here are the opening of the heart centre and the opening of the mind centres to all that is behind and above them. For the heart opens to the psychic being and the mind centres open to the higher consciousness and the nexus between the psychic being and the higher consciousness is the principal means of the siddhi. The first opening is effected by a concentration in the heart, a call to the Divine to manifest within us and through the psychic to take up and lead the whole nature. Aspiration, prayer, bhakti, love, surrender are the main supports of this part of the sadhana—accompanied by a rejection of all that stands in the way of what we aspire for. The second opening is effected by a concentration of the consciousness in the head (afterwards, above it) and an aspiration and call and a sustained will for the descent of the divine Peace, Power, Light, Knowledge, Ananda into the being—the Peace first or the Peace and Force together. Some indeed receive Light first or Ananda first or some sudden pouring down of Knowledge. With some there is first an opening which reveals to them a vast infinite Silence, Force, Light or Bliss above them and afterwards either they ascend to that or these things begin to descend into the lower nature. With others there is either the descent, first into the head, then down to the heart level, then to the navel and below and through the whole body, or else an inexplicable opening— without any sense of descent—of peace, light, wideness or power, or else a horizontal opening into the cosmic consciousness or in a suddenly widened mind an outburst of knowledge. Whatever comes has to be welcomed—for there is no absolute rule for all—but if the peace has not come first, care must be taken not to swell oneself in exultation or lose the balance. The capital movement however is when the Divine force or Shakti, the power of the Mother comes down and takes hold, for then the organisation of the consciousness begins and the larger foundation of the Yoga."

Yoga Sadhana

A LETTER

1. It is not very necessary to study books on Advaita or Dvaita or Vishishtadvaita for practising Yoga. These philosophies have value as presentations of different spiritual experiences of the Reality in terms of the intellect. Each is valid, but from its own standpoint. Each is a view, but not the whole view of the Reality. This is seen when one ceases to merely theorise and speculate and proceeds to realise in experience. As you enter the inner domains of the soul or the higher reaches of the purified mind, the Reality, the Divine, reveals itself not in one aspect, not in one status of itself, but in many. You may start as a Dvaitin, as one approaching Another; and the Divine may suddenly well up deep within you revealing itself as no other than your very own Self. Similarly, the Advaitin may be confronted with the presence of the Beloved around him claiming the adoration of the lover. The fact is the Divine has many aspects, many statuses and that is revealed to the seeker which is most natural to his inner being and most pertinent to his real need, whatever his mental preference.

78

Yoga Sadhana

So it is not at all indispensable that you should study the various philosophies for a successful pursuit of Yoga, though such a study rightly done, can help the mind to enlarge the bounds of its conceptual thinking and to appreciate the multiple character of spiritual experience in its approach to the many-sided Reality that is the Divine.

2. Regarding the experiences : each line of sadhana has its own kind of experiences leading to its definite realisation. The particular state which you describe as 'asamprajnata', where the difference between the seer and the seen fades away and the coiled up energy reaches the thousand-petalled lotus etc., is neither sought after nor normally experienced in the path of the Dvaitin. The Dvaitin would not be disposed to grant the same value to it as the Advaitin does.

Incidentally I may note in passing that 'flashes, blue spots, visions of gods, goddesses and great yogins' are not the only 'early mystical experiences'. These come by when there is an opening of the subtle vision. It may not happen for a long time or at all to many and yet they may well be firmly on the way. Their opening may be at different centres, heart, hearing, mind etc. and their experiences may be of the nature of an onsetting calm or peace, devotion, purity, clarity of knowledge, joy and so on.

3. The visions and experiences you describe are quite genuine. They indicate that you are awake on the subtler levels of existence where these things are usually active; they also show that your being is ready to transcend the normal bounds of physical life and live on its higher ranges. Beyond this it is difficult to say. For each such vision, each experience, is to be weighed and valued in its own context, its background, its results in the waking consciousness. On these planes, there are many entities, benevolent, malevolent and other, and one cannot be too careful against likely masqueradings and enticing misdirections. One thing, however, is certain. If you have a central sincerity in your seeking, then whatever the initial stumblings and errors, the correct meaning and direction will come to you from within or without.

4. Pranayama is no part of the Integral Yoga of Sri Aurobindo though one may practise and use it for purposes of purifying and subtilising the mind, controlling the life-force etc. It can only be a means for a limited end which could well be achieved by less mechanical and more natural means in this Yoga. The period when Sri Aurobindo did Pranayama refers to his early days in Baroda when he practised the traditional Raja Yoga in part and had not yet come to formulate and develop the Yoga which was later built up by him after he came to Pondicherry and took up his spiritual mission exclusively.

5. Re. *Kuṇḍalinī Yoga* :

The signs of the awakening of the Kundalini are unmistakable. There is considerable heat in the body, especially in the region of the Muladhara. Those whose subtle audition is sensitive are said to hear a low droning sound like the murmur of bees when the Kundalini is set active.

When the Kundalini passes through any centre or chakra in its upward ascent, there is a particular experience of bliss at that centre. It is concretely felt and one can know which particular centre has been touched and negotiated. Also one gains a control or the beginnings of a mastery over the *tattva* or principle governed by that centre.

6. Thus far regarding the various queries you have made. Now coming to the most important point in your letter as to what path you should adopt and what discipline you may best follow, the answer is it depends upon your goal in life. And while setting a goal for yourself, it goes without saying that you take into account the equipment with which you are endowed, the nature of your temperament and being, the kind of *saṁskāras* to which your mind is habituated. It is obvious you are not satisfied with the normal type of physical life common in the world. Then, is it a kind of sattvic life governed by the light of the mind and warmth of the soul that you seek ? Or is it a definite turn to the life spiritual ? And if it is a spiritual

career that you choose, do you seek only the salvation of the soul, mukti, or a liberation of the whole
of your being,—the soul, mind, life and body,—
from the hold of Ignorance, and its all-round growth
and fulfilment in the Divine Consciousness with its
essential powers of Knowledge, Will and Joy? If it
is the former, any of the traditional lines of Yoga
may be followed. If the latter then the Integral,
Poorna, Yoga of Sri Aurobindo is the obvious
choice.

You ask what is the practical method of this
Yoga. Put broadly, the Yoga begins with a keen
aspiration for the Truth of life, for the Divine. It
proceeds through a willed opening in the heart, in
the mind and in all the rest of the being to the
Higher Consciousness of the Divine; a rejection of
all that is contrary to the Object of one's seeking;
and a progressive surrender, placing of oneself in
the hands of the Yoga Shakti, the Divine Power
which can be directly received and experienced
through the Grace of the Guru acting through
a look, a word — spoken or written — or in
other innumerable ways. This call and opening
of oneself in consciousness to the Divine Shakti
and the responsive incoming or unveiling of the
Power work out the process of this Yoga which
proceeds in three main movements viz., first, the
realisation of the Divine within oneself; second, the
realisation and identification with the Divine extended in the cosmos; and third, a transformation

of nature leading to a self-transcendence into the
plenary status of Vijnana, the Gnosis.

Thus it will be seen that this discipline is
largely psychological to begin with; it acquires a
spiritual character as it progresses. Physical and
psycho-physical means adopted in other lines of
Yoga could be used here also as feeders to the main
process.

You refer to Sri Aurobindo's remark that this
yoga is the easiest. That is indeed so because it is
the most natural of all yogas inasmuch as it only
concentrates the methods and accelerates the process of Nature in evolution. To grow, to expand
and arrive at an acme of perfection which rejects
no main element that has been evolved but raises
each to its fullest value is the one aim that Nature
pursues in all the million forms of her making and
through her thousandfold processes. The aim of
Sri Aurobindo's Yoga is the same. Only it is not
content to let things develop in the slow, leisurely
motion of the universal Nature. It takes up the
fundamental operation of that Nature, applies it
with a firm and conscious direction in the awakened
being of man and seeks to precipitate within a
single life-time results that would otherwise takes
ages to appear.

Sadhana and the Body

Sri Aurobindo has written : ' Sadhana has to be done in the body, it cannot be done by the soul without the body'. Would it not be easier to do the sadhana when one is relieved of the gross material body and lives in the subtle body alone?

Sadhana cannot be done except with the physical body. The Earth, the Physical is the field of progress, sadhana, evolution. Even the Gods, it is said in the Scriptures, have to come down on the earth, take a physical body and do tapasya if they want to enlarge or exceed themselves. There is no movement of progress on planes other than the physical. Over there things are all set to type and those worlds are content in their typal perfection.

Once you leave the body, the part nearest to the physical, the subtle-physical rushes to find some shelter in some physical abode, in the environs of the family or friends, in trees etc. The rest of the being, the mental and the vital parts clinging to the psychic entity within pass through the intervening planes or stages to the psychic world where the central being rests for recuperation and rest till the

84

time is come for the next incarnation. It does not do sadhana. It simply rests and silently prepares for the coming birth.

Of course there are cases, very very rare though, of persons who after passing away have continued to *live* in the earth-atmosphere, for shorter or longer periods, and exert themselves for the good of those on earth. But they have done so not for sadhana but to make available to all the fruits of their sadhana done during their *life-time on earth, in the physical body.*

The physical ensures a stability, a containing continuity which the other strata of the being cannot provide so naturally to the workings of the Spirit.

Divine Grace and Human Effort

If ultimately one has to depend upon the Divine Grace, what is the necessity of personal effort by meditation, concentration etc. ?

It is true that the Divine Grace is finally the deciding factor. It is quite impossible in spiritual life to effect certain decisive results by human effort alone. It is the intervention and operation of the Grace that precipitates the steps at crucial stages. But there are two sides to this working of the Divine Grace. The manifestation of the Grace is usually preceded by a *state of grace* in the sadhaka. And this state is the slow result of a long preparation and tapasya, whether known to the surface personality of man or not known. Even when the impact of the Grace appears to be sudden we can be sure that there has been ample preparation behind it, either in the present life or in the past.

Not only the manifestation but the working of Grace also has to be supported by human effort. As Sri Aurobindo says, the Divine Grace will act only in the conditions of Truth. The recipient has at every moment to put himself on the side of Truth and reject every element of Un-truth that is foreign to the presence of the Grace. This demands a ceaseless discipline of aspiration, rejection, surrender. The central sincerity has to be spread to all the different parts of the being so as to build a temple of oneself to receive and contain the Divine Grace. Otherwise the Grace recedes.

So human effort is indispensable both prior to the advent and subsequent to the manifestation of the Grace. Tapasya is necessary to invoke the Higher Power. Sadhana is required to receive and keep the gifts of the Grace. Till the higher working is securely established and the charge of the completely consecrated being is taken up by the Divine Shakti, personal effort is essential. The Grace works more rapidly and victoriously in such a responsive and dynamic *ādhāra* than in one given to tamasic resignation and indolence.

Inner Strength and Will-Power

What is the difference between Inner Strength and Will-Power? How to generate and strengthen the Will-Power?

Inner strength refers to the development of the *inner* being of man as distinct from his surface personality which is all he is normally aware of. This inner being consisting of the inner mind, inner vital and the subtle-physical organised round the central being or the soul, carries with it the essence of its evolutionary labour which is reflected in the state of its development, its strength and power as an individual manifestation of the Spirit. This state of the inner being is not dependent on outer circumstances, it exists by itself supporting the further evolution of the soul through the frontal personality. It may or may not be reflected in its fullness in the outer nature which is chosen to suit the purpose for which the particular birth has been taken.

This inner strength, being a developed power of the soul in manifestation, can be increased by the cultivation of higher soul-values and their practice. When so done the inner strength not only gets added nourishment but it comes forward to overtly support and participate in the growth of the evolving person. Otherwise it lies as a reserve behind the activity of the surface elements.

What is normally called will-power is clearly different from this strength. It is a projection in nature of the soul's power for effectuation. Will is the focus of the demand of the being to exist, to live and increase. It is there in the mind, in the life-force, even in the physical body. In some it takes distinct shape and dominates and moulds life as it desires. In others it is incipient and weak, has no power to assert itself, goes under at every opposition and man becomes just a creature of circumstances. But it is possible to build it up into a force for growth and mastery. It has to be cultivated in the way the muscles of the body are developed. One has to activate the will, exercise it deliberately and gradually increase its sway and power. It is easy to sense one's will-element in the mind i.e., in a thought or idea that arises in the mind. If it is a healthy idea, one must make it an occasion to exercise the will and develop it. Pursue the idea, exert yourself to translate it into action. There are likely to be obstructions; but do not give up at the first hurdle. Strive, get over it and proceed to work out the idea. That way the will develops and grows. Similarly if there be a wrong thought or idea, resist the temptation to yield to it. In the very process of thus opposing a move-

ment contrary to the growth of the being, the will
acquires a strength and you will have gained a
larger and stronger fund of will-power for the next
trial of strength. The same holds good on all the
levels of the being, the spiritual, the emotional, the
nervous and the physical. Every circumstance that
presents itself can be utilised for the exercise and
growth of the will-power and consequent development of one's individuality.

As the discipline proceeds, the inner strength
begins to come forward from its depths and express
itself more and more overtly in this will-power
which, ultimately, after its dross of desire and
egoism is burnt away in the fire of tapasya, trans-
forms itself into a pure dynamis of the soul.

Law of Karma

You have stated[1] that the powerful man who exerts himself prospers whatever his moral deserts whereas his virtuous competitor lacking the requisite will-power fails to make good. Why is it so?

This statement has been made while discussing the Law of Karma and its manifold working. Karma means that a given output of energy calls back the same energy in the form of a result. The energy that flows back is commensurate with the quality and the quantity of the output. The nature of what is put forth decides the nature of what comes in consequence. Thus if a certain effort is made in the moral direction the result too will be on the moral plane. A moral discipline for instance will promote a moral strength and increase the moral courage. Its results are not to be sought for in material terms. For results in the material sphere, exertion has got to be on the material level. Thus a moral effort will produce a moral effect, a spiritual effort produce a spiritual result and an output of force in the physical economy of things

[1] *Sri Aurobindo : Studies in the Light of His Thought,* p. 54.

91

produce results in a physical way. This in brief is the doctrine of Karma in pure theory. In practice, however, the fact that man lives and acts simultaneously on several planes of existence introduces a complicating factor of the interaction of their several movements. There is also the factor of the Karma of the environment, the Karma or heredity etc. But to return to the question.

It is clear why success or failure in the material field is not dependent on the moral qualifications of a man. It depends mainly on the energies poured out in the material way, the labour that goes into the physical working. Goodness or badness of the doer has little to do with the matter. For moral excellence there is a moral consequence, not material advancement. Each line of Karma is different from the other and an output in one should not be confused with results in another flowing from a cause in their own kind.

Meditation

I begin to get thoughts in the mind the moment I sit for meditation. However much I may try they do not stop and even after half an hour of effort I do not get more than a minute of peace and quiet. There is an exhaustion at the end. How long should the exertion be made? How to quiet the mind?

It is not that thoughts begin to come in when one meditates. Thoughts are there all the time, only one does not normally take notice of them as one is occupied with something or the other. When one begins to meditate, all the mental faculties are withdrawn from outer activities and one gets aware of the movement of thoughts some of which come from outside and some appear to rise from within. To struggle with them and sit upon them is not always the best method. Keeping a central remembrance of the purpose for which one is sitting, one can let the thoughts run their course; only one must keep to the remembrance taking care not to run with the thoughts. One does not succeed immediately, but there should be a patient and persistent come-back to the main Thought every time there is a sliding into the running current of thought-activity. In course of time the thoughts dwindle.

Another method is to put a will and concentrate or gather the consciousness round the object of meditation ignoring the existence of other thoughts. Aids like Japa or visualisation of an image or a felt invocation to the Divine Person who embodies the object of your seeking, may be used to draw the mind from its running course and still the thought-movement. If you cannot centre the mind around the object of meditation immediately, keep it centred in a circle closely related to that object. Foreign movements will automatically recede for want of supporting attention.

In any case there should be no strain. To learn to relax and release the consciousness in a flow on the object of seeking is the secret of meditation. Reading of elevating literature, recitation of a few rhythmic passages from scriptures for a little while, create a helpful background for meditation.

It is hard to quiet the mind by one's own effort. The easier way is to remember and conceive of a Silence, a Quiet that is there behind everything, behind your mind, and call upon the Silence to enter into you. If done with faith there is bound to be a response, sooner or later, and then you have only to let yourself into the folds of the Quiet or the Silence that comes in an enveloping movement.

Disturbing Thoughts

Whenever anyone known to me is reported to be ill or starts out on a journey, I get inauspicious thoughts. What is to be done on such occasions?

Usually it is attachment or some kind of self-interest that gives rise to such apprehensions, *atisnehah pāpas'anki.* At the root of such movement is a fear on the part of the ego that it may lose a support. It may also be that such thoughts and fears are drawn to itself by a nature or a mind which is habitually morbid and constantly dwells on the wrong side of things. There are, in the present constitution of the universe, a number of beings and forces which embody dark movements like anxiety, fear, terror etc. and they are always on the look out for likely receptacles for their activities. The only way to counter their invasion is to resolutely shut them out, refuse to look at them much less entertain them. It is difficult but it has to be done in some form or the other. This is a negative way of rejection. The positive way is to place reliance on the Divine and every time such thoughts and fears come in, to refer them or surrender them to the Divine and yourself remain trustfully quiet. After all nobody is going to be helped by your entertaining these apprehensions. If at all, by giving a mental body to these amorphous ideas you help them in their attempt to effectuate themselves and thus cause indirect injury to those for whom you profess concern. On the other hand if you remember the Divine on such occasions there is a double advantage: the wrong suggestions melt away before the Light which you invoke and you do not give them a chance to formulate themselves in shape: a helpful vibration is set going for the benefit of the person concerned.

Sadhana and Apparel

I have a liking for bright colours in clothes. As a sadhika, is it desirable for me to avoid wearing such clothes as they may attract other people's attention which might affect my consciousness? Should I cease taking interest in such dresses?

There is nothing at all wrong or unspiritual in wearing bright or beautiful clothes. Beauty is an important part of the Divine Manifestation and it is a kind of perverse denial to refuse to participate in that movement. As much as Knowledge, Power and Joy, Beauty also—with all its picturesque variety—is a facet of God to be manifested in each individual, even as it is abundantly manifest in Nature on all the planes of existence.

The question about attracting other people's attention is a little more complicated. There it is really a matter which depends upon oneself. If there is no intention of drawing attention from outside, in however concealed a form, then, as a rule no such attention is drawn. Whatever attention may be directed from others would not be of such a nature as to produce vibrations of consequence in your consciousness. It is usually when something in you wants and waits for it that there is an impact of that kind. It does not matter what you wear or do not wear. But it does matter why you wear it. To look pretty or beautiful is not unspiritual or immoral. But to embellish oneself in order to provoke admiration or invite attention, consciously or subconsciously, is not very wholesome for one's wellbeing.

Sadhana and Gifts

Can a sadhak accept gifts from others? Will there not be an exchange of undesirable vital forces? What should a sadhak do if forced to accept gifts by relatives?

Naturally, a gift always carries with it something of the person who gives it. It may be goodwill, affection, sentiment of regard or devotion. It may also be a claim subtly laid on the recipient. At its worst it can be a physical means to establish a relation with the receiver for any purpose, nefarious or otherwise.

It follows that it is the spirit accompanying the present that should determine the right course —to accept or not to accept. In ordinary social life it is indeed difficult to refuse gifts from friends, relatives etc. And the obligation that ensues on accepting a present is usually offset by a return-present in due time. Where however, the recipient is not in a position to return, the obligation remains; a vital claim is established and his freedom of movement in his relations with the giver is compromised to that extent. In spiritual life, luckily, it is not incumbent on the sadhaka to conform to this social convention of gifts. He can impose on himself a wholesome discipline of not accepting any presents at all; or if he is obliged to accept by special circumstances, he should inwardly offer it to the Divine within and accept on His behalf. Thereby he saves himself from the consequences of the gift.

Sadhana in the Ashram

It is said that in the past sadhaks had had several experiences in their sadhana which they do not get these days. Why? Is it that the method of working of the Mother has changed? Or is it a necessary stage in the collective sadhana?

In a collective life like the Ashram, there are certain dominant factors which stamp themselves on the consciousness of the constituting members. The most important of these is the working of the Yoga-Shakti of Sri Aurobindo and the Mother. The central feature of its workings is always reflected in the inner life of the inmates whether all are conscious of it or not. That is why during the earlier years when the Mother was working upon the mental and vital planes subjecting them to the pressure of the descending Power, sadhaks here used to experience so much activity in the inner layers of their mind and vitality. Visions, voices, inrushes of knowledge, power, joy—all these experiences were the indices of the stir of the general movement in the mental and vital layers of the collectivity. As the work was completed, as far as could be, on these

101

SADHANA

planes, the emphasis was shifted to the subtle-physical and physical planes and for the past one decade or more, the Mother has been directing the Yoga-Force on the physical and below the physical. These layers are denser than those of mind or life regions and naturally the results of the pressure thereon take time to express themselves in the *ādhāras* of individuals, especially if they are not particularly attentive and responsive.

Comparatively speaking, the response was readier and more spectacular in the mental and the vital parts of the collective being for the reason that they are subtler by nature and nearer the spirit in the gradation of Existence. Besides, the aspiration and preparation of the sadhaks was more adequate in these parts than it has been in the physical. Even so, it is not that there are no experiences now. Experiences there are, only they are not of the kind people were used to. Those who are sensitive do see the results of the impact of the Higher Force and Consciousness on the physical system, specially the stronger resistance of the body to the forces of disintegration, greater resilience in responding to touches of the Mother's Force and so on.

Movements Outside and the Ashram

There are spiritual movements (like that of Unity people in Missouri) which often speak and preach and believe in what the Mother believes, believe in some sort of a new and better world for which the time is now ripe, and emphasise on the spiritual meaning of religion; their whole approach to all personal and other problems is spiritual. But they are not consciously in touch with the Mother. No doubt it must be the New Force that is at work. But would it make any difference to them if they turned consciously towards the Mother? I mean in the process of their transformation, in the realisation etc.

When new truths begin to descend into the earth atmosphere there are many who receive them. But each grasps and formulates according to the nature and competence of the mind that perceives. Some receive them fragmentarily, some in a fuller measure. It is only the rare few, in fact those who can be said to be born to embody and manifest these truths, that see them whole and express them adequately. Now, the Ideal of a perfect life on earth, the vision of a New Age of God-men has been there for a long time and it has been glimpsed and promulgated in inspired utterances by several men in several communities and various efforts have been made to translate them in actual life. But rarely have any two such movements been identical. Their language may appear to be very much the same but there is always a difference in their import and their application.

Coming to the matter in question, though there are today a number of movements aiming to prepare and equip for a new life of harmony, peace and unity, their objectives, methods and their whole outlook on life are radically different from those of the Teaching and Yoga of Sri Aurobindo and the Mother. 'Spiritual movements', like the one you speak of, have the betterment of the human lot as their aim. Reduction of stress and strain, amelioration of conditions, increasing happiness and security in life are what they generally have in view. To this end they draw upon or adapt the tenets of one religion or another or formulate some sort of a system combining the fundamentals of all religions with an element of occult practice. But our endeavour is set in a totally different key. We do Yoga not for human ends, however laudable, but for a Divine Purpose and this Purpose includes a radical, not piecemeal, change of the human nature into its ultimate term of super-nature—a real transformation of the whole of the living man which is not envisaged elsewhere. The Divine has willed that a higher Consciousness shall manifest and lift up the entire life in creation to a new dimension. The Mother embodies the Power that works the Will and She has chosen some from humanity who are prepared to surrender themselves to the Call of the Divine and make themselves its instruments for the reception, manifestation and establishment of the New Consciousness.

Naturally though the immediate field of the Mother's direction of the New Consciousness-Force that is now manifesting, its physical centre, is the Ashram community, the range of its influence is wider and in course of time the whole earth will come under its Glory. Meanwhile—till this divine Power of Knowledge-Will gets into its full stride and begins to function on an organised basis—all progressive movements working for the elevation of man, for the clearance of the backwaters of Ignorance, darkness and misery, receive and will continue to receive an indirect help and impetus from the Force centrally acting through the person of the Mother. It goes without saying that if any individual or movement turned directly to Her and received inspiration and guidance immediately from Her that would make a tremendous difference. It does make a difference whether you stand directly below a shower or are content to receive the distant spray.

Gayatri

There is a popular belief that the Sri Gayatri mantra is not very responsive to the spiritual aspirant in this Yuga. But I am attracted by that Mantra and have been doing its japa. I am of the view that the Light that is invoked in the Gayatri Mantra is the supramental Light and the aim is supramentalisation. Is that correct?

I am not aware of any such popular belief regarding the incompatibility of the Gayatri with spiritual life in this age or any other. On the other hand in almost all upāsanās, Vaidic as well as Tantric, there is a Gayatri addressed to the Devata that is adored. Possibly the claim made in the *stutipāṭhas* (laudatory stanzas) of the Mantra that it promotes all the four traditional aims of life, *dharma, artha, kāma* and *mokṣa,* may have given rise to the belief that since other interests also are served by the Mantra it is to that extent inimical to true spiritual ends.

In these matters it is as a rule safe to welcome a Mantra for which one feels some attraction, on practising which one feels happy. It is a friendly Mantra which has affinity with something in you.

I am not sure that the aim of the Gayatri is supramentalisation; I rather think it is not. This

much is certain : the Sun that is addressed is not
the solar orb in the sky but the Sun of Spiritual
Truth at the head of creation whose symbol in this
universe is the physical sun. The Light that flows
from that Sun is the illumined energy of the creative
Consciousness that is massed therein. The Vaidic
Gayatri (of Rishi Vishwamitra) prays for the acti-
vation of one's intelligence by the rays of that Light.
A spiritual illumination of the mind, the highest
evolved part of man is what is sought for. And this
is indispensable in all spiritual disciplines that
proceed through an awakening and growth in the
Way of Jnana, Knowledge of the Divine, though
it may not be very relevant for the Way of Bhakti.

Supramentalisation is far different and much
more. It implies the lighting up of not only the
mind but the whole of one's being, not merely rendering it luminous with knowledge but charging it in
other ways of being also viz., feeling, will, action
etc. so as to transform the human nature into the
Divine. That is the aim of Sri Aurobindo's Gayatri
which runs :

*Tat savitur varam rūpam jyotiḥ parasya
dhīmahi, yannaḥ satyena dīpayet.*

Let us meditate on the most auspicious (best)
form of Savitri, on the Light of the Supreme which
shall illumine us with the Truth.

OTHER TITLES BY SRI M.P. PANDIT:

Bases of Tantra Sadhana	2.00
Commentaries on the Mother's Ministry, Vol. I	6.95
Commentaries on the Mother's Ministry, Vol. II	7.95
Commentaries on the Mother's Ministry, Vol. III	14.95
Dhyana (Meditation)	1.95
Dictionary of Sri Aurobindo's Yoga	7.95
Gems from the Veda	3.95
How Do I Begin?	2.95
Occult Lines Behind Life	3.95
Spiritual Life: Theory & Practice	7.95
Yoga for the Modern Man	4.00
YOGA OF LOVE	3.95
YOGA OF SELF PERFECTION	7.95
YOGA OF WORKS	7.95
YOGA OF KNOWLEDGE	7.95

available from your local bookseller or

LOTUS LIGHT PUBLICATIONS
P.O. Box 2, Wilmot, WI 53192 U.S.A.
(414) 862-2395